REIKI HEALING FOR BEGINNERS

Your Step-by-Step Guide to Mastering Reiki in 21 Days

By Karen Gray

TABLE OF CONTENTS

INTRODUCTION

Reiki is a system of natural healing, originating in Japan, that employs universal life energy. This tradition was started by Mikao Usui in the early twentieth century. It focuses on the energy surrounding us, flowing through us, affecting everything. When this energy flows harmoniously, without interruption, we feel a sense of well-being.

Reiki treatments can provide emotional and spiritual help for your body, and is open to any belief system. It can be used alone or with other complementary or conventional treatments.

The experience of Reiki is different for every individual, depending on their needs at the time, but some **benefits reported by different people** are:

- Deep relaxation
- A strong sense of calm
- Well-being
- Heat
- Tingling
- Color
- Emotional response

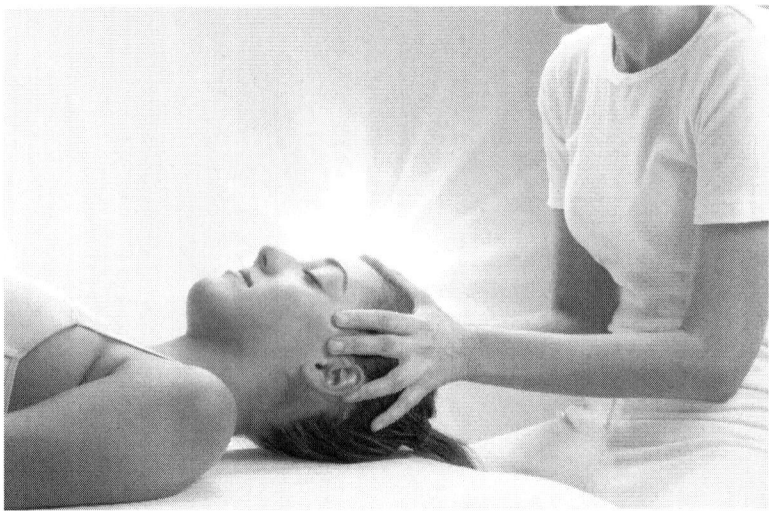

This book will provide you with all the different aspects and techniques that support Reiki Healing. Within the following chapters, you will learn about the history, practice, training, and effects of the treatment, and how to apply it to your everyday life.

Not only will you receive advice on picking the right practitioner, you will also learn how you can help yourself and other people with Reiki principles and practices. You can also gain the magical ability to become a spiritual doctor. By the end of your reading, you will have a complete guide to energy and well-being, success, and healing with Reiki.

So, read on for a step-by-step guide for how to learn and use Reiki to heal yourself and others, including the very important guided meditations. Find your own well-being and lead a more harmonious life.

HISTORY OF REIKI HEALING

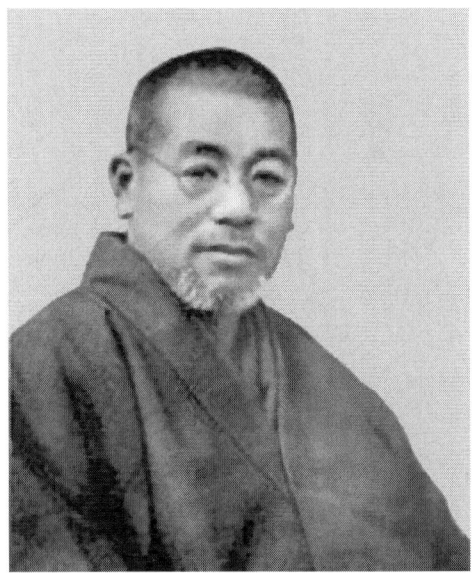

Reiki Healing was founded by Dr. Mikao Usui, who was born in 1865 and grew up in a wealthy Buddhist family. He received a great education because of his family's money, and through this, he developed an interest in medicine, psychology, and theology.

He wanted to find a way to self-heal that wasn't attached to any specific religious belief so it would be accessible to everyone. To follow this belief, he traveled a lot through his lifetime, studying all kinds of healing around the world.

Eventually, he stopped traveling and joined the Buddhist monastery. During this period, he attended a rediscovery training in Mount Kurama, where he spent 21 days fasting, meditating, and praying. On the twenty-first day, Usui's life was changed when he saw the ancient Sanskrit symbols, which led to him believe that the key to healing was in the laying on of hands.

Reiki spread quickly; with Usui opening a clinic and school in Tokyo in 1922, teaching others his techniques. These students, notably ex-naval officer Dr. Chujiro Hayashi, developed the techniques even further.

One particular patient, Mrs. Takata, is believed to be the person who brought Reiki to the West. She got sick and needed surgery, while traveling in Japan in 1935, but didn't want to use traditional medication. She used and fell in love with Reiki, eventually becoming a Reiki Master herself and spreading the healing to America.

How Does Reiki Work?

Although not every Reiki session is the same, there are some standard practices. The recipient remains clothed during the session, which will typically last at least 45 minutes, and at most 1.5 hours, depending on the recipient's needs. During the session, the healer will gently place their hands on, or nearby, the recipient's body in a series of non-intrusive areas.

This works because of the life force flowing through and around the body, nourishing the organs, and supporting vital functions. It flows through using pathways called chakras, meridians, and nadis, and is using the aura energy that flows around us.

Disrupting this force diminishes the function of organs and tissues and encourages negative thoughts and feelings.

Reiki heals the weakened areas of your energy field, infusing them with positive energy. It vibrates and breaks up the negative energy so it falls away.

Is There Any Proof?

For a while, Reiki was looked down on in the same way that other complementary treatments have been, so scientific studies weren't conducted. The first recorded evidence-based study, which was made available to holistic, medical, and scientific communities in 2005, was conducted by William Lee Rand. Rand is the president, and founder, of the *International Center for Reiki Training*.

This study (*ncbi.nlm.nih.gov/pubmed/20706088*) became known as the **Touchstone Process** and rigorously critiqued the best Reiki practices. It's known for its intensive, impartial look at everything Reiki.

The most recent data recorded in this shows strong evidence supporting how Reiki promotes a positive biological response, particularly when it comes to stress, anxiety, depression, and pain levels.

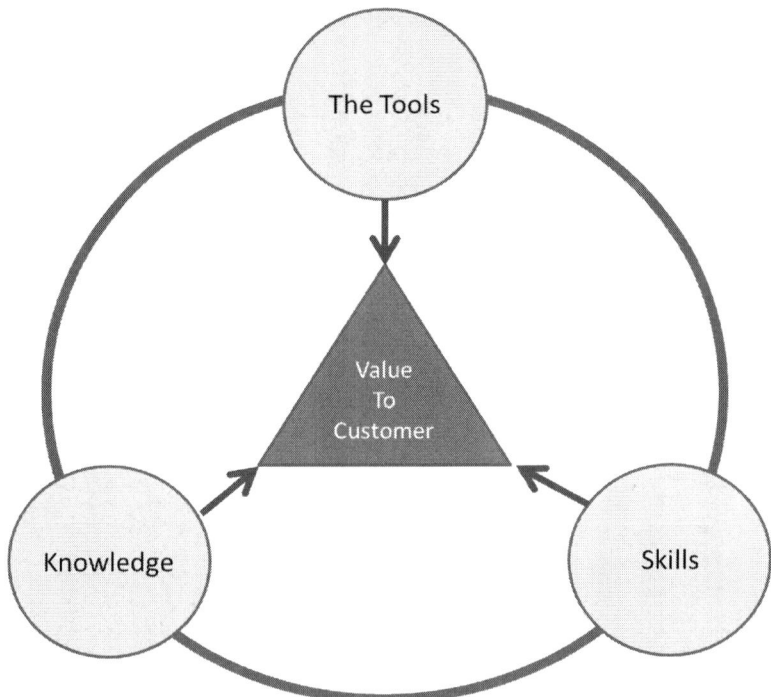

The Touchstone Method

Another study was conducted by Columbia University and New York Presbyterian Hospital to prove how effective Reiki treatments are for the **autonomic nervous system**. This blind random study showed results in heart rate, respiration, and blood pressure.

Other studies (at *thehealingpages.com/benefits-of-reiki-in-hospitals*) have shown **Reiki is effective for**:

- Pain after a tooth extraction
- Cognition in dementia and Alzheimer's patients
- Relaxation for pre-op
- Pain for post-op
- Pain for chronic illness
- Depression and stress
- Well-being

A research study at Hartford Hospital
(at *dahlc.mayoclinic.org/2015/12/29/9-facts-about-reiki*) found:

- 78% of patients experienced reduced pain
- 80% of patients experienced reduced nausea
- 86% of patients experienced improved sleep
- 94% of patients experienced reduced anxiety during pregnancy

Some of the **more in-depth studies into Reiki** and specific diseases, which have had positive results, include:

- ***Reiki experiences of women who have cancer*** *(at ncbi.nlm.nih.gov/pubmed/27119403)* An exploratory study from 2016 had findings suggesting that Reiki has benefits as a tool for women with cancer to self-manage quality of life issues.

- ***Effect of Reiki on patients who have total knee arthroplasty*** *(at ncbi.nlm.nih.gov/pubmed/26760383)* Pilot study from 2016 showed decreased pain ratings and positive feedback following Reiki sessions. So much so, a Reiki program was established at the hospital where ten nurses trained to become certified in Reiki.

- ***Reiki and massage to reduce anxiety and stress*** *(at ncbi.nlm.nih.gov/pubmed/27901219)* Random clinical trial from 2016 showed Reiki and massage produced better results in reducing anxiety and stress among the subjects.

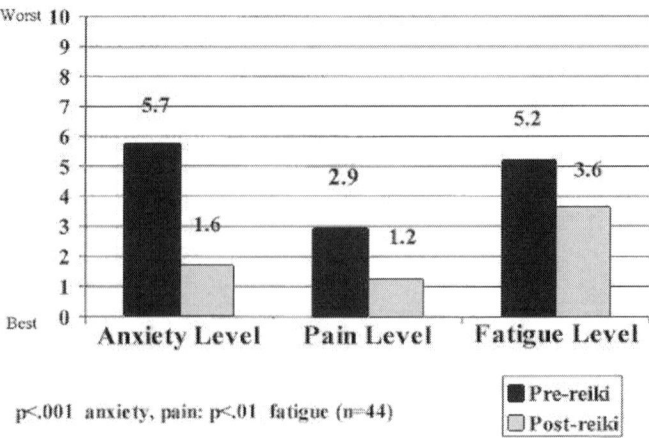

p<.001 anxiety, pain: p<.01 fatigue (n=44)

All of this is very positive. The more scientific studies that are conducted, the more positive outcomes will be discovered.

Who Is It For?

Reiki is for everyone. Everyone has the ability to channel Reiki; it just needs to be activated. Since it promotes well-being in the whole body and isn't designed for specific illnesses, everyone can gain some benefit from it. In this busy world with lots of stress, everyone could use a sense of relaxation and calm.

To gain the benefits of Reiki, you can either visit a practitioner or learn to do it yourself. Many people find self-care the most effective way. Depending on how much effort you wish to put into it, you can go all the way to Reiki Master.

Reiki provides solid benefits for anxiety and depression, alleviating the 'fight or flight' response and generating a better sense of calm. It's also helpful for reducing the side effects of several health and chronic conditions, such as long-term pain and migraines and headaches, by strengthening the immune system.

What Are the Benefits of Reiki?

Here is a list of many **benefits of Reiki**, which can give you an idea of how this healing can help improve your life:

- *Harmony and balance* – mental and emotional balance in the left and right side of the brain can be achieved by enhancing the body's natural healing ability.
- *Relaxation* – Reiki helps to release stress and tension from the body.
- *Dissolving energy blocks* – promoting the natural flow of energy.
- *Supporting the immune system* – cleansing toxins from the body.
- *Grounding* – clearing the mind and helping you to feel centered.
- *Rest* – better sleep equals a clearer brain.
- *Self-healing* – Reiki helps the body return to its natural state.
- *Pain* – the promotion of self-healing alleviates pain.
- *Spiritual growth* – emotional cleansing.

Why Was There Ever Doubt?

Despite all the proof found in studies, there are still **some common misconceptions about Reiki**. But these are just myths and don't affect how well it works at all:

- *Religion* – a lot of people believe that it's linked to religious beliefs, which isn't the case at all.

- *Spiritualism* – there is a worry that Reiki is linked to the spiritual world, but again this isn't the truth.

- *Massage* – Reiki isn't massage therapy. It can be used alongside manipulation, but they are separate treatments.

- *Energy* – giving Reiki to others doesn't diminish your own energy. The energies used in Reiki don't ever run out.

- *Healing* – the Reiki practitioner doesn't heal you directly, but rather gives your body the tools it needs to heal itself.

- *One-Time* – Reiki isn't a one-time thing; it's an ongoing process if you want to get the most from it.

- *Complicated* – Reiki is a simpler process than it looks.

TEN SURPRISING FACTS ABOUT REIKI

You may think you know everything that you need to about Reiki, but **here are some facts that might still surprise you!**

1. Reiki isn't just for humans. Animals, plants, food, and water can also benefit.
2. Reiki is incorporated into patient services in over 800 hospitals.
3. Reiki energy can be sent at a distance, anywhere in the world.
4. Reiki can also be sent and programmed for a time in the future.
5. There is a limitless source to Reiki energy. It won't run out.
6. Once the Reiki energy is flowing, you don't need to concentrate. You can carry on with your day, while the magic is working.
7. Reiki isn't just about healing. It can also help you develop inner knowledge and feel more in control of your life.
8. During the 9/11 disaster, a Reiki station was established to treat the responding firefighters and paramedics.
9. Many Reiki practitioners work with professional sports teams to aid recovery and to enhance performance.
10. Reiki treats all glands and organs.

FIVE KEY REIKI PRINCIPLES

Dr. Mikao Usui developed five key principles for practitioners to live by on a daily basis, to help fully embody the energy. The idea behind these principles promotes well-being and can be useful to anyone. Even for those who do not have an interest in Reiki, these ideals are good to live by. They invite happiness into your life.

"Just for today, I will not worry."

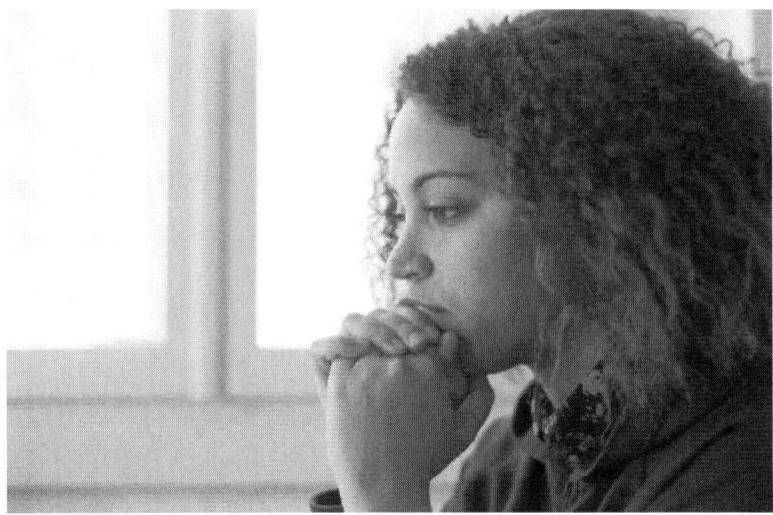

Stress is a major issue for most people. Daily lives, balancing careers and family, finances, social lives – dealing with everything that life throws at us is very problematic and has a very negative impact on us. It can cause headaches, insomnia, heart issues, and digestive problems to name just a few. Since a study (at *mentalhealth.org.uk/statistics/mental-health-statistics-stress*) showed that 74% of people have felt so stressed they feel unable to cope in the last year, we can see what a massive issue this is.

Most of the things we are stressed about cannot easily be changed. Worrying about it certainly doesn't have a positive effect. It just makes things worse.

This needs to change.

It can feel impossible to think that you won't be stressed anymore, but *"just for today, I will not worry"* is achievable and is a great way to start.

"Just for today, I will not be angry."

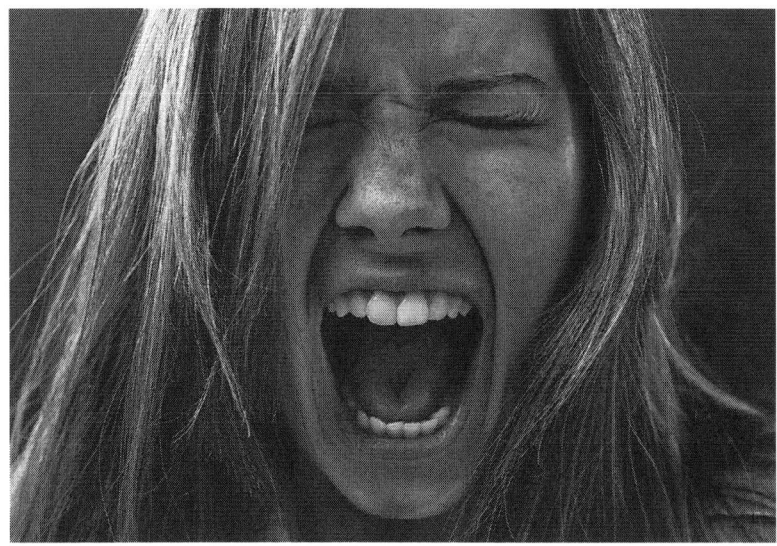

Anger is often a default emotion that we fly to when things don't quite go our way. There's no coffee in the morning, a driver cuts you off in the road, your computer fails – it makes you feel angry before anything else, which isn't good for your health. It can also cause headaches and high blood pressure, which can lead to long-term issues.

A study (at *angermanage.co.uk/anger-statistics*) has shown that one in ten people feel like their anger is out of control, with 64% of people thinking that people, in general, are getting angrier.

If you feel like anger is a real issue in your life, then it's best to seek professional help before it takes over your life, but if this is just a small issue, then just for today, every time you feel that familiar anger bubbling, try taking a deep breath, counting to ten, and letting it go.

See how good you feel at the end of the day.

"Just for today, I will be grateful."

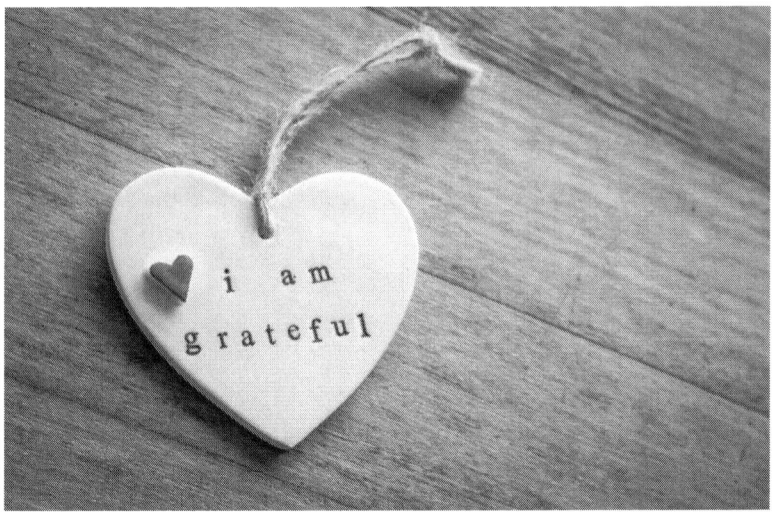

It's human nature to want what we don't have. To yearn for other things in life. But this isn't helpful. A scientific study has shown that **gratitude has proven benefits**:

- The laws of attraction show that gratitude opens the doors to more relationships. People will want to be nearer to you.

- It improves physical health because your well-being is improved.

- It gets rid of toxic emotions, improving your mental health and strength.

- Empathy is enhanced, aggression is reduced, as shown by a study conducted by the University of Kentucky (at *forbes.com/colleges/university-of-kentucky*)

- Better sleep is achieved by those who are grateful.

- Gratitude also helps improve self-esteem.

So, why not, just for today, try being glad for what you have. Whether this is a job, a car, a house, a family, health, friends – whatever it is, be positive about it and smile.

"Just for today, I will do my work honestly."

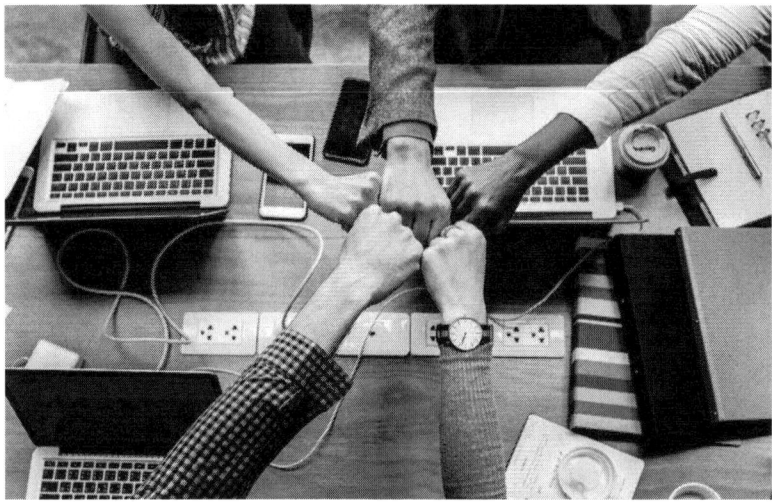

Working honestly brings a sense of purpose and meaning. It's tempting to skate through each day, but that leaves it feeling a bit like a waste of time. Give it a try, just for today, and see how fulfilled you feel at the end of the day.

"Just for today, I will be kind to every living thing."

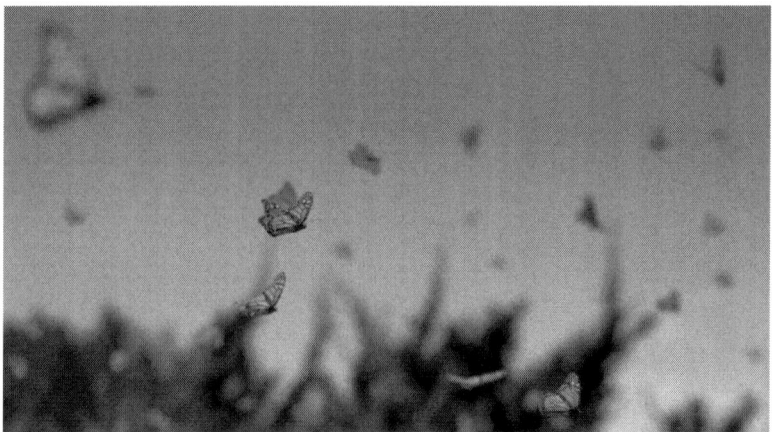

Give love and kindness to anything and anyone who crosses your path to-day and see what benefits you receive. It's true that whatever you put out into the world is what you get back, so give it a try. Act with compassion, bring light into someone else's day, if even for a moment, and see what you get back.

If these principles seem overwhelming to try all at once, focus on one each day to see how it makes you feel. Eventually, you can apply them all to live a happier life.

INITIATION

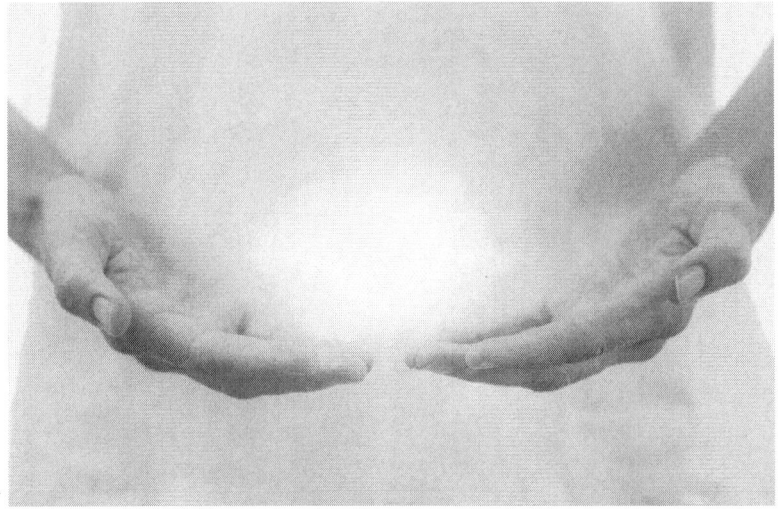

The Reiki initiation, often known as an '*Attunement*,' is the process of starting with Reiki and activating your inner energy via a ceremony. You can read about Reiki and learn about positioning, but until you have an Attunement with a Reiki Master, you cannot truly practice it.

As the Reiki Master passes down the skills to the student, allowing them to become a vessel, it's a powerful spiritual experience. Your pathways are opened, and the Reiki energy can easily flow through your body. Many report feeling weightlessness to their body and tingling sensations all over.

To become a Reiki Master, a person requires three levels of training, which will be discussed in more detail later. How long each level of training lasts will depend on how well you adapt and where you receive training. The process can be as short as a few hours or last as long as a few years. Each level can be achieved in just one session each or be spread out over a few sessions. It can vary.

Someone who has already achieved Reiki Master status will guide these sessions, where you will be correctly attuned. An online search can help you find a Reiki Master near you.

What Happens?

The Reiki instructor will touch the student's head, shoulders, and hands, using special breathing techniques to help the energy flow into the student. This is important because the energy pathways are fully opened, allowing the Reiki energy to flow forever. Without it, the Reiki will not fully work.

This is just the first step of becoming a Reiki Master, but it's an important one. After the Attunement, many people like to go through a 21-day cleanse to help rid the body of negative energies, emotional blockages and to promote healing physically, emotionally, and spiritually. This involves giving yourself a Reiki treatment for a minimum of 40 minutes every single day over 21 days.

This can lead to negative emotions coming up, often referred to as the 'healing crisis,' which can be a bad time. Not everyone experiences this, but if you do, just remember that it's your body getting rid of toxins.

Reiki Levels

There are three levels of practicing Reiki. The Attunement and cleansing process are **Level 1.** If you only want to use the Reiki energy for yourself, then this will be enough, but for many, they want to also share their magic with others, so move on to Level 2.

Level 2 allows students to receive the Reiki symbols (which we will discuss later in this book) and receive another attunement. The teachings will be about opening up to more energies, working on others, and also distance Reiki.

Level 3 turns you into a Reiki Master, able to pass on the energies to another person. This usually happens after some time, once a deep commitment to Reiki has been demonstrated.

Choosing the right practitioner to guide you through all of this is very important. You want to be comfortable to get the most out of it. The first thing to look for is accreditations. If they belong to a Reiki society, then chances are, they take it much more seriously, and the second thing to do is talk to them. Ask questions, find out more, then you can decide if you have the same goals as them.

The Three Reiki Pillars

When starting Reiki, you will be taught about **the three pillars**. These help you to meditate using Reiki energies. They are also very important for treating others with Reiki. There are three parts to this, *Gassho*, *Reiji-Ho*, and *Chiryo*, and each is important on this new self-healing journey.

Gassho

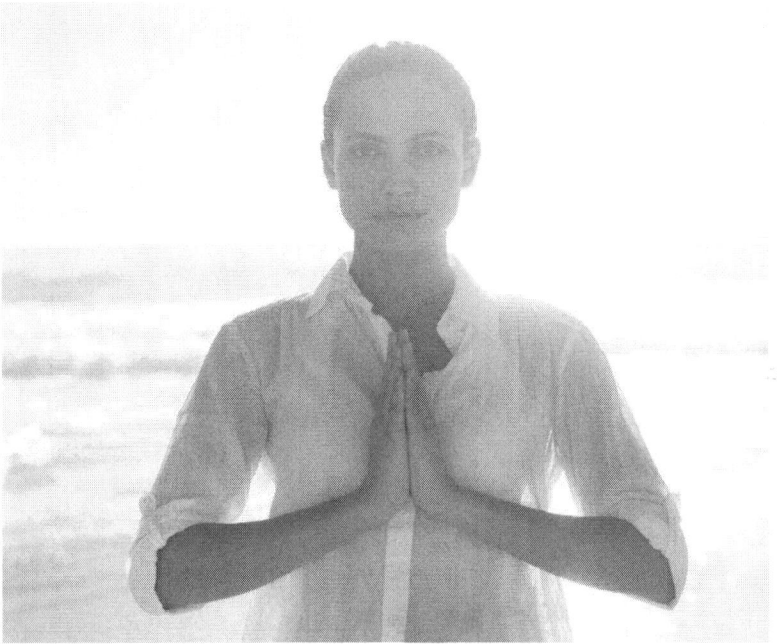

Gassho is the first pillar, which means 'two hands coming together.' It focuses on respect, focus, balance, gratitude, and connection.

To achieve this pillar, place your hands together in a prayer position, while meditating, and bring your awareness to the tips of your middle fingers. Recite the five Reiki principles and send out the intention of gratitude.

It's best to perform this in the morning for 15-30 minutes for one month.

Reiji-Ho

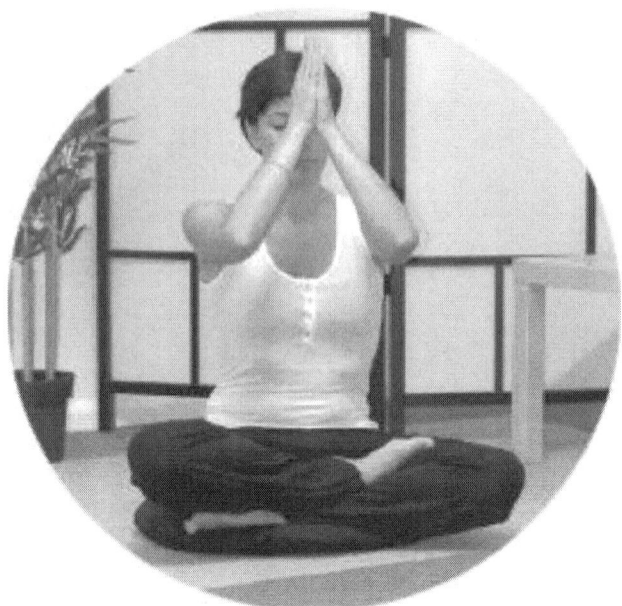

The second pillar focuses on Reiki power and consists of three short rituals to be performed before each session. *Reiji* is Japanese for 'indication of Reiki power,' and *Ho* is translated to 'method.'

- Put your hands in the Gassho position in front of your heart. Then, with your eyes closed, ask for the Reiki energy to flow through you.

- Then ask for the well-being of the recipient. Raise your hands to your third eye and ask for guidance as to where the Reiki energy is needed.

- Allow your hands to be guided, forgetting your own desires for the session. Trust your intuition.

Chiryo

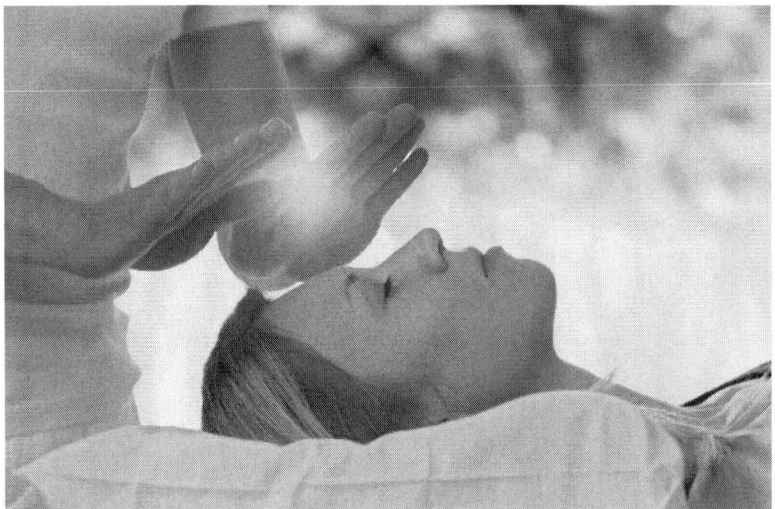

This means 'treatment' and involves the practitioner holding their dominant hand above the crown of the client's head and waiting for a signal to move. Follow your intuition until the session comes to an end.

There are some people who talk about self-attunement; it is increasingly being considered just as effective as traditional methods. You will need to be very familiar with the symbols for this, and extremely self-controlled, but it's considered possible.

ALL YOU NEED TO KNOW ABOUT REIKI ENERGETIC SYSTEM

The Reiki energetic system works from **three places in the body**. Working with these, starting with these whenever you face an issue, can help balance yourself to face anything.

These are:

Earth Energy (*Hara* – below the navel about 3 inches (8 cm), the core of everything according to Usui.)

When the term hara is mentioned, it references the "lower" hara. The symbolic energetic center for *Earth Ki* (life force or energy that flows through everything). Within that center, original energy is stored. This energy is the essence of your life, energy you were born with, and provides your life's purpose. This original energy is a direct connection between you and the universal life force, and it is not just the energy you received from your parents at your conception.

Heavenly Energy

This is a symbolic energetic center holding *Heaven Ki*. This energy is directly connected to your spirit. If you are connected to this center, you might see colors or experience psychic ability. It is important to stay centered and not become unbalanced. Using this energy in a balanced way will allow you to see beyond the immediate.

Heart Energy

This is a symbolic energetic center holding *Heart Ki*. Energy from this center is connected to emotions. This is 'human' energy that is connected to human experience. You can understand your life's process through this center – from childhood to adulthood and back to childhood. As a child, you lack experience, but as you grow, you turn into a child with experience.

All of these energies are important, particularly when it comes to Reiki. Being in tune with them can help you to use them to your advantage. Especially, when considered with the five elements and seven chakras that we will go on to look at through the rest of this chapter.

Five Elements

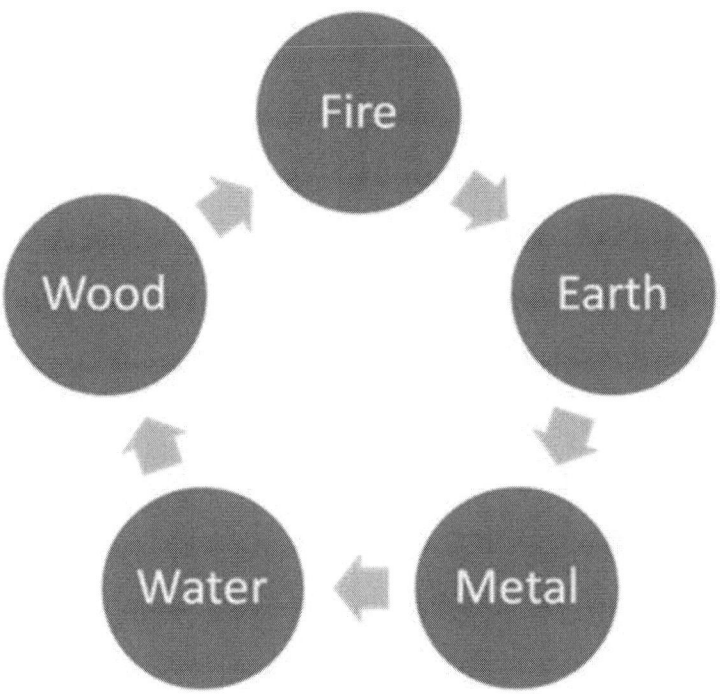

Five element Reiki focuses on the **five main elements**: Wood, Fire, Earth, Metal, and Water. This is not to be taken literally, but is more about the qualities that these elements embody. Each element works in its own way, but they all need each other and to work in harmony to be effective.

5 Element Reiki (at *5elementreiki.com/about/five-element-theory-chi*) has a good explanation of this:

"Water creates Wood by nourishing it. Wood feeds Fire by being fuel, Fire produces Earth as ash through combustion, Earth produces Metal as minerals, and Metal feeds Water by becoming condensed essential fluid (Earth's core is molten iron, mercury is liquid at lower temperatures, for example). Then, the process repeats with a new set of conditions."

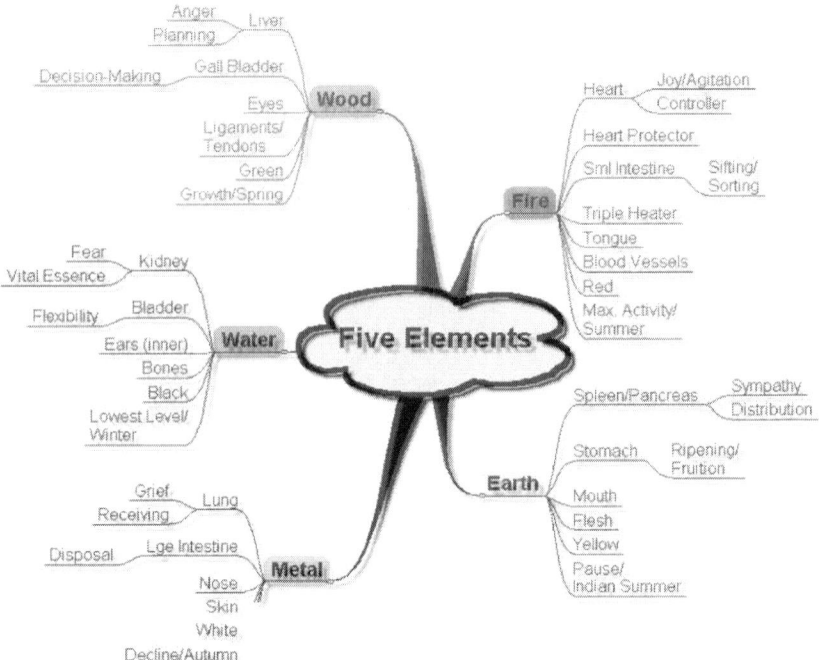

By applying these elements to the body, they relate to Reiki very well:

Wood

Wood represents the eyes. Any issues with eyes can be linked to an imbalance in the liver or gallbladder, headaches, and aggression. Vision issues can lead to poor decision-making, which is why we need to keep it balanced.

Fire

Fire represents the ears, heart, and small intestine. The heart protector is associated with hearing, and the small intestine is associated with sound, so this is all linked. A fire imbalance makes it difficult to listen to others.

The tongue is also represented by fire, so any speech impediment is linked.

Keeping a balance with fire and water is incredibly important.

Earth

This element is represented by the flesh. Connective tissues and fat tissue. A wasting disease is down to an imbalance in the earth element. The mouth, stomach, and spleen are also linked.

Ideas are associated with the earth, so if someone is having trouble creating ideas, then this imbalance may be why.

Metal

The nose is linked to metal, and because of this, so are the lungs, the large intestine, and mucus. Any breathing issues or funny smells is a metal imbalance. The skin is also linked.

The best time of day to help conquer a metal imbalance is between 3:00 and 7:00 a.m.

Water

Water is represented by our kidneys. But it's also linked to our willpower, survival instinct, and sex drive. Issues with it can be seen in kidney stones, kidney and urinary tract infections, bone diseases, loss of hair, some types of watery diarrhea, menstrual disorders, insomnia, and constantly cold hands and feet.

The best time of day to deal with these issues is between 3:00 and 7:00 p.m.

To live our best life, all of these elements need to be working at their best, and working in harmony as well. Seeing the signs for an imbalance in any elemental area gives a practitioner a clear idea of what work needs to be done.

Seven Chakras

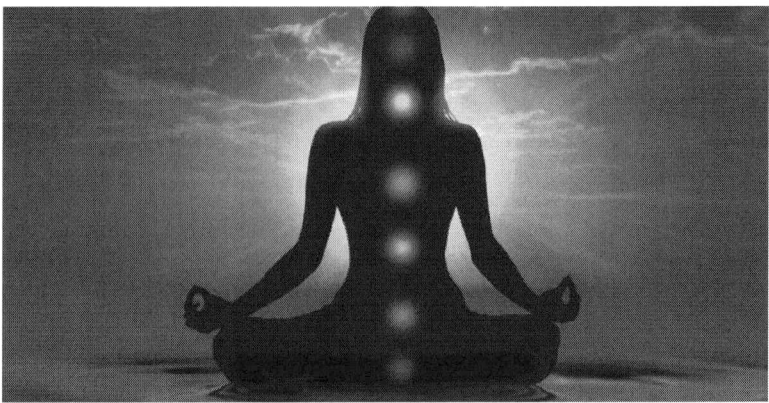

The word *'chakra'* might seem like a newer concept, but it actually dates back to 600-2000 BC. It's also associated with Yoga as well as Reiki. Chakras are concentrated centers of energy in the body that are designed to keep us functioning at optimum levels.

The seven chakras are associated with positive well-being and correspond to the nerve ganglia directly, which are attached to the spinal column. The chakra positions relate to the endocrine glands, which secrete directly into your bloodstream, and are associated with an organ or bodily function.

They are centers of energy inside the human body that link to emotions, behaviors, and feelings. So, when these are blocked, there are issues that follow.

The **seven chakras are located**:

1. Base of your spine
2. Lower back and abdomen
3. Between navel and sternum (solar plexus)
4. Heart
5. Throat
6. Between eyebrows
7. Crown of your head

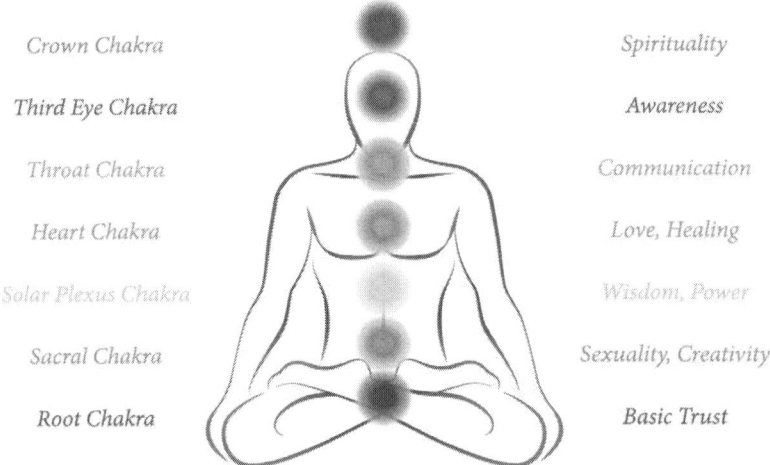

Crown Chakra	Spirituality
Third Eye Chakra	Awareness
Throat Chakra	Communication
Heart Chakra	Love, Healing
Solar Plexus Chakra	Wisdom, Power
Sacral Chakra	Sexuality, Creativity
Root Chakra	Basic Trust

These are often associated with colors as well, as shown in the diagram above. The chakras in the lower part of our body link to basic instincts, and the higher ones govern our thoughts, behaviors, and characteristics.

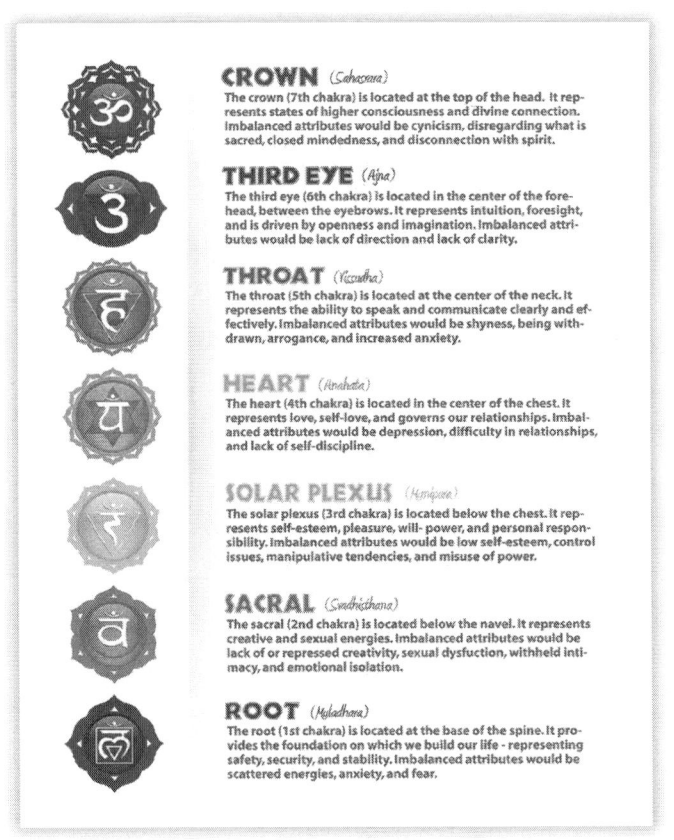

CROWN (Sahasrara)
The crown (7th chakra) is located at the top of the head. It represents states of higher consciousness and divine connection. Imbalanced attributes would be cynicism, disregarding what is sacred, closed mindedness, and disconnection with spirit.

THIRD EYE (Ajna)
The third eye (6th chakra) is located in the center of the forehead, between the eyebrows. It represents intuition, foresight, and is driven by openness and imagination. Imbalanced attributes would be lack of direction and lack of clarity.

THROAT (Vissudha)
The throat (5th chakra) is located at the center of the neck. It represents the ability to speak and communicate clearly and effectively. Imbalanced attributes would be shyness, being withdrawn, arrogance, and increased anxiety.

HEART (Anahata)
The heart (4th chakra) is located in the center of the chest. It represents love, self-love, and governs our relationships. Imbalanced attributes would be depression, difficulty in relationships, and lack of self-discipline.

SOLAR PLEXUS (Manipura)
The solar plexus (3rd chakra) is located below the chest. It represents self-esteem, pleasure, will- power, and personal responsibility. Imbalanced attributes would be low self-esteem, control issues, manipulative tendencies, and misuse of power.

SACRAL (Svadhisthana)
The sacral (2nd chakra) is located below the navel. It represents creative and sexual energies. Imbalanced attributes would be lack of or repressed creativity, sexual dysfuction, withheld intimacy, and emotional isolation.

ROOT (Muladhara)
The root (1st chakra) is located at the base of the spine. It provides the foundation on which we build our life - representing safety, security, and stability. Imbalanced attributes would be scattered energies, anxiety, and fear.

So, now that you know where the chakras are, we're going to look at **how to feel them**. It may not happen right away, but if this is important to you, then you should keep trying until you do:

- Start with finding a quiet peaceful place to sit with your eyes closed. Take a few deep breaths and let any stress fall away.

- Focus on your body; start at the base of your spine and imagine a spinning red light there. Sit with that feeling for a while.

- Move your attention up a little closer to your belly button and feel the warm orange light there. Feel it move with your breath.

- Now focus on the area just above your belly button and sense the intense yellow light.

- When you reach your heart, the light becomes green. You can place your hand on your heart to really connect.

- Move to the dip in your throat. It's bright blue. If you need to swallow, then do so.

- Head to your eyebrows and your third eye. As the indigo light flashes there, you become wiser.

- At the top of your head, the spinning light is violet. This light connects you to the universe.

For further reading on this subject, check out the *Mind Valley Blog* at <u>*blog.mindvalley.com/7-chakras*</u>.

Keeping your chakras balanced and making sure everything remains harmonious inside the body can be done in a number of ways, including:

- Reiki
- Massage
- Yoga
- Meditation
- Exercises
- Holistic Medicine.

A lot of these suggestions are things that you can do alone to balance your chakras. It isn't something that you need to visit someone else for, which is great news, because a blockage can be very problematic for you.

Here is **an exercise you can practice** to get you started:

- Put yourself in the mind-set, or energy state, of the emotion you desire. Start by letting go of expectations of, especially those, or attachments to, the outcome of this exercise.

- Bring your knees up, putting your feet flat on the surface beneath you, while you lie on your back. Inhale through your nose, then breathe out through your mouth. Be sure to relax your jaw.

- Think of your breath expanding your belly just like a balloon. When you exhale, squeeze your Kegel muscles and flatten your lower back against the surface beneath you. There will be a gentle rocking of your pelvis as you breathe.

- Imagine pulling energy from your root chakra – the base of your spine – as you breathe in. The energy will follow your thoughts; you won't have to push or pull.

- Inhale, moving your energy from the root chakra to the sacral chakra. As you exhale, the energy circulates back to the root chakra. Keep moving this energy between the chakras by inhaling and feeling it rise to the sacral, then exhaling and letting it drop to the root. Repeat, and you will notice the energy moves easily – nearly on its own.

- You can enlarge the circle you've established by breathing healing energy up to your solar plexus chakra. Squeeze your Kegels as you exhale. Repeat this, as well. When you feel this is complete, shrink the circle to send the energy between your solar plexus and sacral chakra.

- Keep breathing and squeezing your Kegels as you enlarge this circle of energy to move from your sacral chakra to your heart. When you feel this is complete, shrink the circle to send the energy between your heart chakra and solar plexus. This is moving the energy from sacral to heart, then solar plexus to heart.

- Now make two circles of energy; one, between the solar plexus and throat, and two, a small circle between throat and heart. Vocalize when you reach the throat if you aren't already doing so, for example, sighs or moans, even "oohs." This helps to create a deeper chakra healing and move energy. As the momentum builds, energy circles may start moving through the chakras on their own.

- Inhale to move energy up from the heart chakra to your third eye, and exhale to move energy down to the heart chakra. Repeat this, followed by creating a small circle between the third eye and throat chakras. Roll your eyes up as you send energy into your third eye, but keep them closed – imagine you can see out of the top of your head. This helps your energy rise and your chakras to heal and achieve balance.

- Your next energy circle moves from the throat to the crown chakra, which is followed by a small circle formed between your third eye and crown chakras.

- Continue breathing and rocking your hips to move the energy in circles, giving your body the space to go through the full process of chakra healing and energy body rejuvenation.

Healing and keeping these balanced is a great way to overcome the demands of everyday life. Stress is unavoidable, and it puts a strain on our energies that leaves us blocked and risks illness, whether that be mental or physical.

Insider Tips

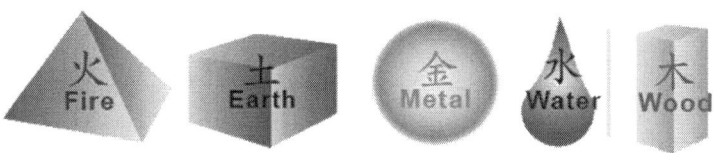

Here are some **tips to help you determine if your chakras are blocked**:

Root (Red, the base of your spine, Earth)

- You feel sluggish.
- Stress is unrelenting because of a reliance on external circumstances.
- Your career and finances are less than ideal.
- You have abandonment issues.
- You have a strong self-hate.

You need to work on getting this open to have better communication and a deeper openness with the people in your life.

Sacral (Orange, below your belly button, Water)

- You struggle with sexual intimacy.
- You feel abused, and that sex will be painful.
- You move from one relationship to another, searching for love.

Healthy sexual experiences are important to life, and a block in this chakra cuts off a very powerful energy inside of you.

Solar Plexus (Yellow, above your belly button, Fire)

- You feel powerless and like a victim.
- You give power away to try and maintain relationships.
- You struggle to achieve your goals.
- You suffer from anxiety and stomach pains.

You need to unblock this chakra to regain your power so you can live a more successful, fulfilling life.

Heart (Green, center of your chest, Air)

- Fear of commitment.
- You have high walls so you don't get hurt by love *again*.
- You struggle with love and compassion.
- You hold grudges.
- Your weak heart chakra can lead to heart disease, asthma, and allergies.

Finding comfort in relationships and giving love means you will receive it much more easily. Your life will feel much lighter with this chakra unblocked.

Throat (Blue, bottom of the neck, Sound)

- Fear of speaking up and expressing how you feel.
- You go along with others, even if it makes you uncomfortable, which leaves you frustrated.
- You often have a sore or blocked throat.

Speaking your truth is freeing, and having it heard is even better. Reiki can be wonderful for helping with this chakra.

Third Eye (Indigo, between your eyebrows, Light)

- You feel disconnected from life and struggle to find any meaning.
- You have trouble with decision-making, particularly when it comes to your spiritual path.
- You feel frustrated and get a lot of tension headaches.

You need confidence in your life's path to get any kind of satisfaction from your existence. Clearing this blockage will benefit you greatly.

Crown (Violet, top of the head, Thought)

- You feel lonely, insignificant, meaningless.
- You disconnect from your spiritual self and connect to material possessions instead.
- You suffer from migraines and tension headaches.

Unblock this to gain an immense gratitude towards yourself and your life. This will also reconnect you to spirituality.

Proven Tips to Transform Negative Energy

To purify the negative energy in your life and to transform it into something more positive, here are some suggestions that work not just on you, but on the life that surrounds you:

- Declutter – the mess in your house can accumulate stagnant energy and block the flow. It's amazing how getting rid of clutter can help clear out the mind.

- Smudge – burn sage, lavender, or cedar as you walk through the house to clear out the negative energy.

- Reiki – the symbols can also help clear out any negative energy.

- Crystals – clear quartz, black tourmaline, and amber are great for purifying bad energy.

- Salt – salt baths or a salt lump can transform negative energy.

Reiki can remove blockages that have been hindering you, which makes it particularly helpful in transforming negative energy and keeping energy flowing smoothly. Positive intention alongside the healing energy in the Master's hands can remove negative energy, even negative emotions and thoughts, to leave you feeling lighter.

YOUR STEP-BY-STEP GUIDE TO GETTING STARTED WITH REIKI

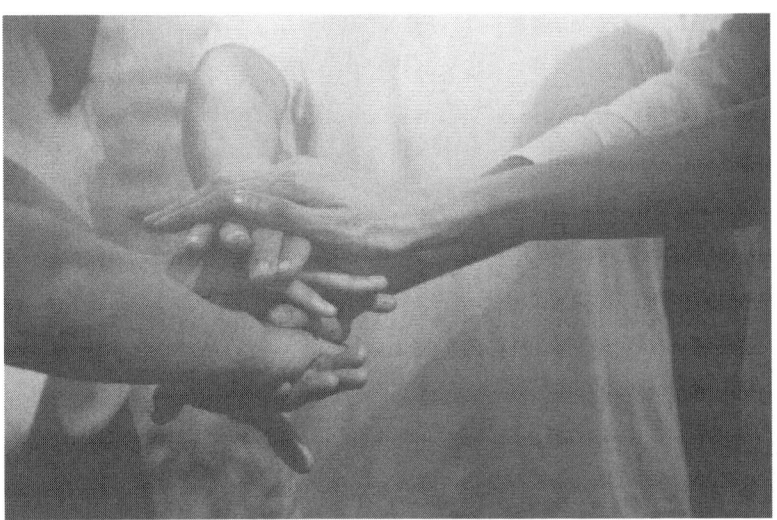

This chapter will look at **what you need to get you started with Reiki**. Even if you are a beginner with absolutely no knowledge, there is nothing holding you back. This energy can be activated by anyone, no matter what your age, skills, or knowledge.

What do I do during a treatment?

It's best to begin with actually having a treatment, to see how it makes you feel. You cannot be sure that Reiki is for you if you haven't experienced it. An online search will let you know where you can make this happen in your area.

Here is a great **step-by-step guide for a Reiki session**, which can be particularly useful when going in for the first time.

Before:

- Eat and hydrate a few hours before the session so you're comfortable and not distracted.
- Relax and reflect for at least 30 minutes before you go in. Notice physical sensations, thoughts, and emotions.
- Use the restroom, again, so you aren't distracted.
- Get comfy for your session.

During:

- The practitioner will talk to you about what is going to happen and to discover what is going on with you to ensure this treatment will be effective. The practitioner may ask what is bothering you, if you are aware of any current blockages, what you've tried in the past, and the status of your physical sensations and emotions.
- You will lie or sit comfortably.
- The practitioner will place their hands on or near your body to get the energy flowing. You may feel the energy flowing through you as this happens. IARP (*iarp.org/reiki-sensations*) suggests that *"you may feel heat, warmth, cold, subtleness, steadfastness, or forcefulness,"* and also that *"Reiki works like a thermostat that regulates the body. Much like a furnace that automatically turns on and off to regulate the temperature, Reiki flows slowly or rapidly – as needed – to dispense balancing energies. Like a pendulum swinging back and forth, Reiki sometimes moves erratically, other times smoothly. These fluctuations of ki energy churning within us can often be felt as pins-and-needles tingling, hot flashes, goose bumps, chills, throbbing, etc."*
- Then, the practitioner will ask you more questions in order to determine the effect this session had on you. Both of you may revisit feelings or sensations from the beginning of the session to discuss what subsequent sessions will entail.

After:

- Take 15 to 20 minutes after the session to consider everything that's come up in the session. Meditate or walk in nature.
- Hydrate and eat to replenish your body.
- Reflect and contact the practitioner if you need to.

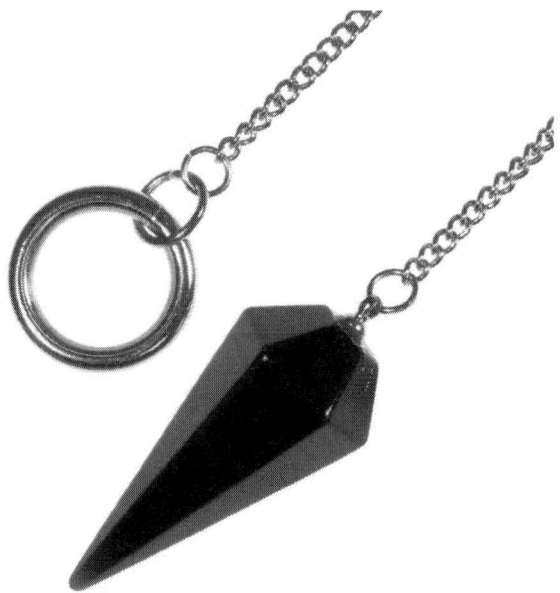

Reiki practitioners often use **pendulums** – wood, crystal, or glass – during the healing. Regardless of what the pendulum is made of, each medium has specific healing qualities and can absorb energy. Pendulums work in harmony with Reiki by clearing blockages in chakras and picking up on the body's subtle vibrations.

Pendulums are held above each chakra and used to find out how the energy is within that area. If it's healthy, the pendulum will move in a clockwise circle. If not, it will move in another direction, alerting the healer to the issue.

How do I do it?

Once you have experienced Reiki, you may want to think about learning it yourself, but you have to confirm that you're ready first. Here are some **signs that suggest if you're ready to move on to the next stage**. This could be right away or after a few treatments:

- You love yourself and appreciate everyone else – healing comes from within, and that's even more true if you're a practitioner. You need to expand your energy to help the rest of the world, so you need to start from a good place.

- You believe in the power of alternate healing – while conventional medicine has its place, you also value yoga, acupuncture, and complementary medicine.

- The unexplained isn't an issue – you welcome the energy of others, you sense or see auras, you feel benefits from crystals.

- You trust in the universe's energy and its power.

- You're ready for a change.

You are then ready to start going through the stages of attunement where you will activate your own energy and begin to help yourself and others. You will learn the traditional hand positions and also how to observe energy to see where help is most needed.

Because **Reiki practitioners are often asked to help with various things**, the treatments are always different. This can include:

- Pain

- Anxiety

- Nausea

- Side effects of medication

- Support after an injury or surgery

- Insomnia or broken sleep

So, you may need to adjust your treatments accordingly, but the **basic hand positions to transfer Reiki energy**, which you will become accustomed to for self-treatment and treating others, are:

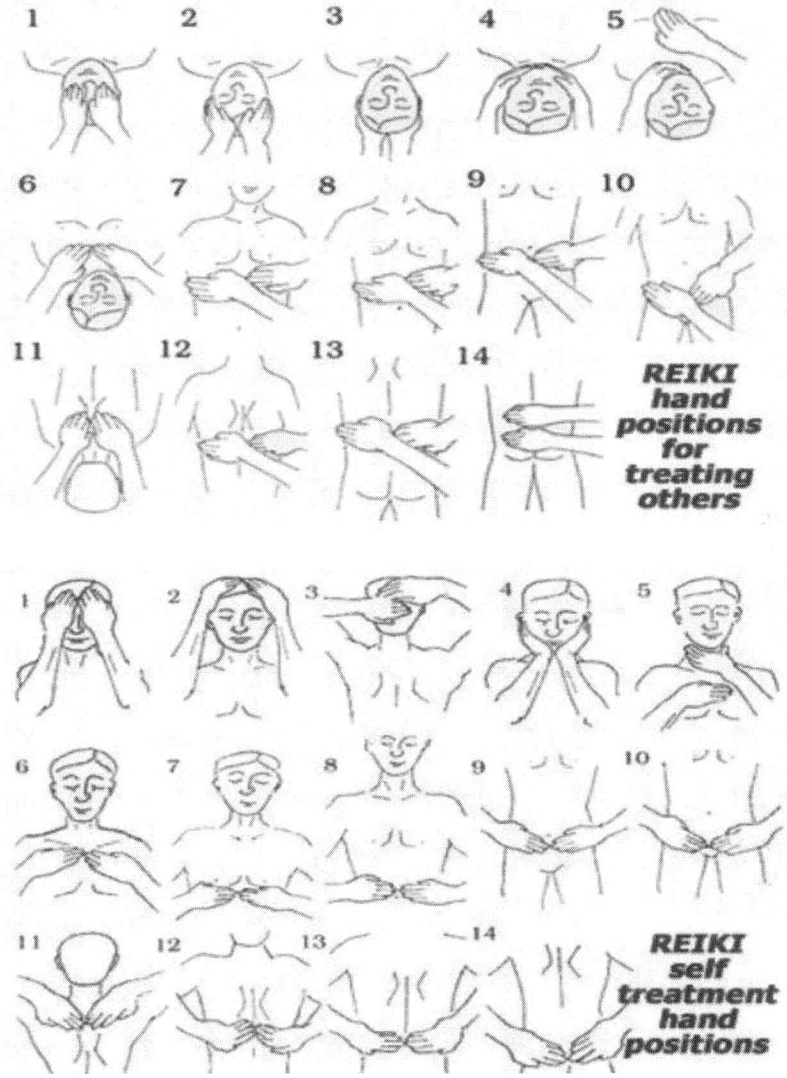

For further reading on this, check out *The Reiki Page* at *thereikipage.com/handpos.html*.

As suggested before, this **can be adjusted according to what the receiver needs**, as shown by this guide below:

Ailment: Eye problems, asthma, stress, headaches, sinuses, gland issues, scribal nerves.

Hand Position: Cup your hand and gently rest them over your eyes, cheekbones, and forehead.

Chakra: Third eye.

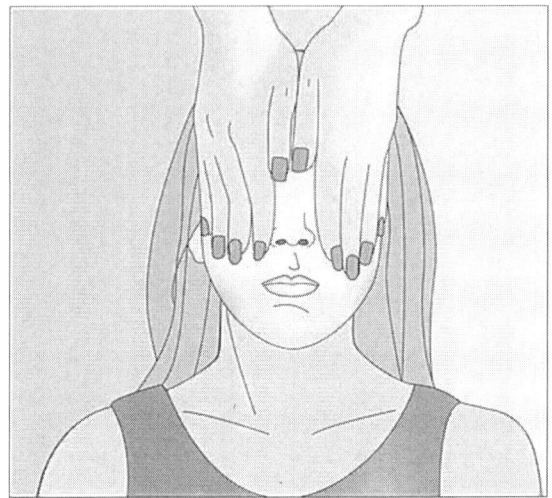

Ailment: Migraines, headaches, eye problems, multiple sclerosis, stress, bladder issues, digestive disorders, emotional problems.

Hand Position: Place your hands on the top of the head.

Chakra: Crown.

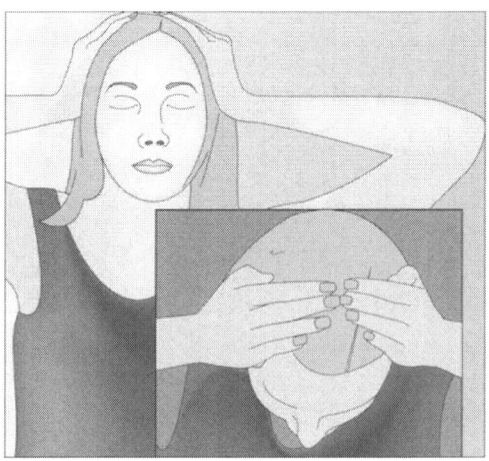

Ailment: Balance, cold or flu, tinnitus, ear problems.

Hand Position: Hands on either side of your head with fingers covering your temples.

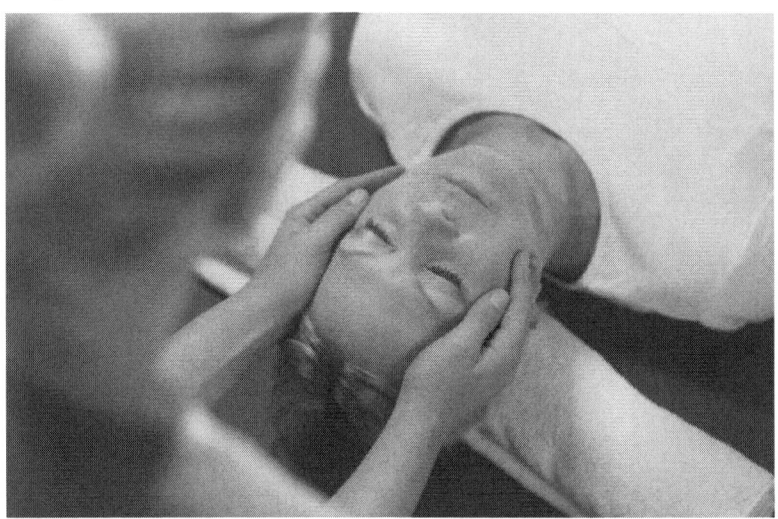

Ailment: Headache, eye problems, stress, fever, sinuses, digestive disorder, phobia, shock, fear.

Hand Position: Place your hand at the back of your head, covering the occipital ridge.

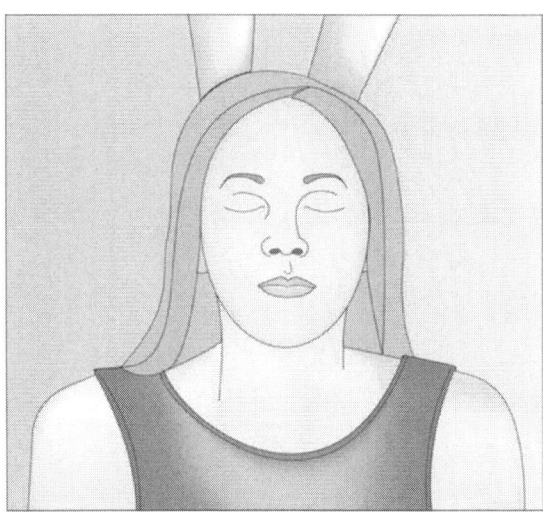

Ailment: Neck and spinal problems, nerves, stress.

Hand Position: Hands covering the top of the shoulders and bottom of the neck.

Chakra: Throat.

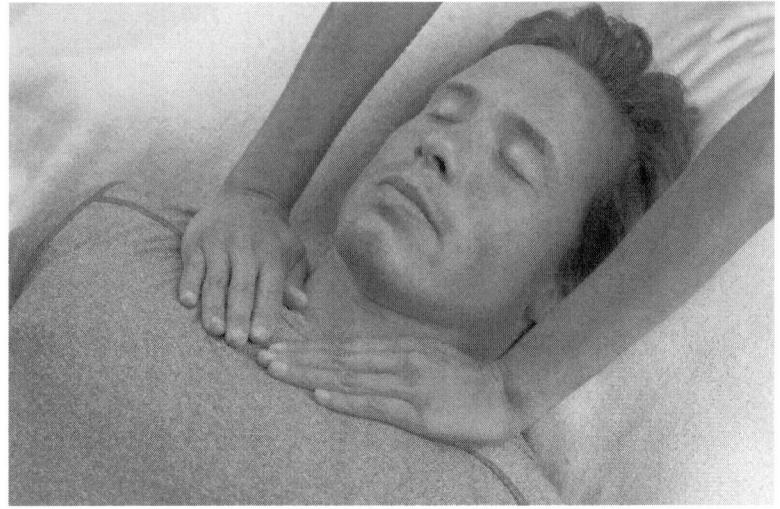

Ailment: Self-expression, communication, breathing, speech problem, bronchitis, flu.

Hand Position: Place your hands with the heels covering the throat.

Chakra: Throat.

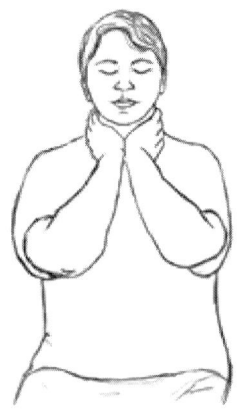

Ailment: Lungs, thymus, thyroid, immune system, emotional problems, and stress.

Hand Position: Hands forming the T; the left hand would be on heart chakra, and the right hand would be on thymus gland.

Chakra: Heart.

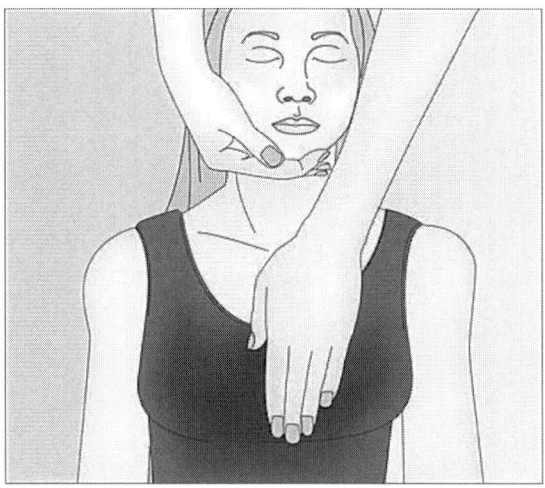

Ailment: Intestine issues, reproductive problems, stomach, digestive system issues, infection.

Hand Position: Hands are placed horizontally at the top of the torso with fingers touching; move hands down over solar plexus, then over the navel, finally ending in a V inside hip bone.

Chakra: Heart, Solar Plexus, Sacral.

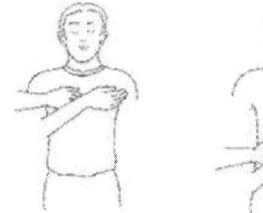 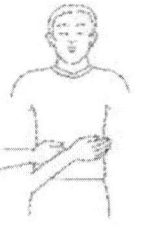 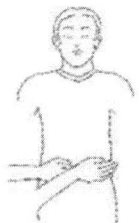 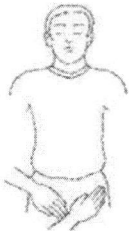

Ailment: Leg pains, veins, circulation.

Hand Position: Place hands over the front of the knees.

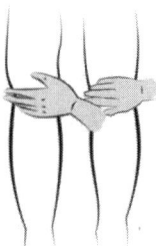

Ailment: Back issues, spinal problems, stress.

Hand Position: Hands are positioned at the back of the shoulders, gradually moving down horizontally across the back, ending in a V at the base of the spine.

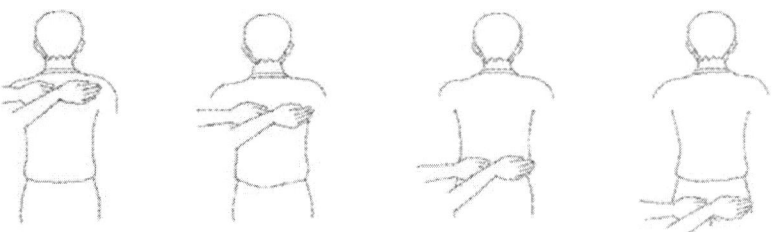

How do I use Reiki?

Reiki can be used for more than just healing yourself and other people. There are many **interesting and creative ways in which you can use this energy** including:

- A bubble – visualize a person you would like to send Reiki to and when you'd like them to receive it. Imagine a colored bubble of love around it, depending on what you'd like the Reiki to achieve (i.e., pink for love, blue for calm, etc.). Channel this bubble for five to ten minutes, then send the bubble.

- Empower your food – yes, you can send the energy into your kitchen to create a more harmonious place, but you can also channel it into the food to enhance what you're going to eat. Say: *"Reiki on: I receive the nutrients my body needs from this meal, for the highest and greatest good of all life and soul, with ease and grace"*.

- Charge something important – your crystals to get the most healing energy out of them, a child's toy, a treasured possession – anything can gain benefit.

- Help your plants – place your hands over the plant or hold the pot and channel the energy. You'll be surprised about how well this works!

- Ease conflict – do not try to impose will or dictate an outcome; simply channel your Reiki energy into a difficult situation to ease it.

- Empower affirmations – end by saying *'for the highest good of all'* for maximum benefit.

- Help fertility – practice during every day of the conception process for best results.

- Burns and bites – the pain can be eased with Reiki.

- Problem-solving – this could be anything from bigger life problems, to simply technology not working as you want. A clearer mind leads to better solutions.

- Use a pendulum to assist you in Reiki and energy healing.

- To help with daily worry – chant the following to help you: *"Reiki on: I know there is a solution; Reiki on: I know there will be a perfect time; Reiki on: I know there are resources available; Reiki on: I focus on what I can work with"*.

The more you practice, the stronger and more effective your Reiki energy will become. This includes attunements. Of course, when starting out, it's important to have a guide to start this process, but once you are more of an expert, you can do **self-attunements** when you would like to strengthen yourself.

Here is **a step-by-step guide** for this:

- Sit down in the middle of a room, preferably on a comfortable chair.
- Include an affirmation that this will be a self-attunement to refine your Reiki and prepare as normal.
- Stand, imagining that you are leaving your astral body in the chair.
- Move behind the chair and give your astral body, still in the chair, the first attunement.
- Continue around to the front and finish the attunement process.
- Include the final blessing.
- Sit back down, returning to your astral body.
- Meditate and focus on the new energy you feel.

Who can help me?

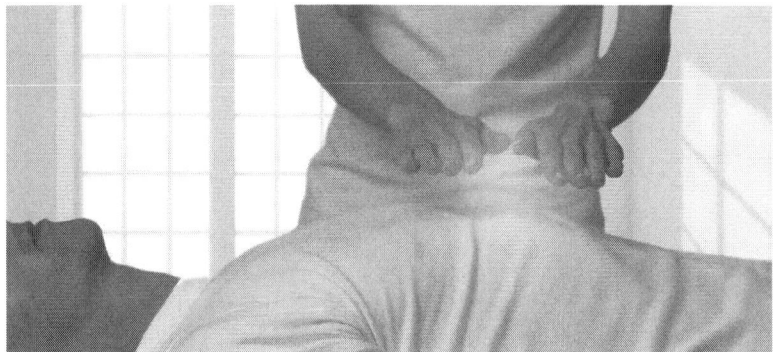

As said before, while you can self-attune, it's better to begin with a guide, especially if this is something that you have absolutely no experience with. That way, you can experience Reiki, learn all about it from someone with a lot of knowledge, and ask any questions you think of along the way. You can also experience the passing on of energy in the attunement.

When looking for a guide who suits you, there are **some things you should consider**:

- How long has the person been practicing?
- What associations are they involved with?
- How often are the classes, and are they affordable to you?
- What will you learn?
- Will you gain accreditation?

A great place to start for this can be *Reiki Fed* (*www.reikifed.co.uk*), *Reiki Association* (*reikiassociation.net/home.php*), and *Reiki Council* (*reikicouncil.org.uk*).

What do I need?

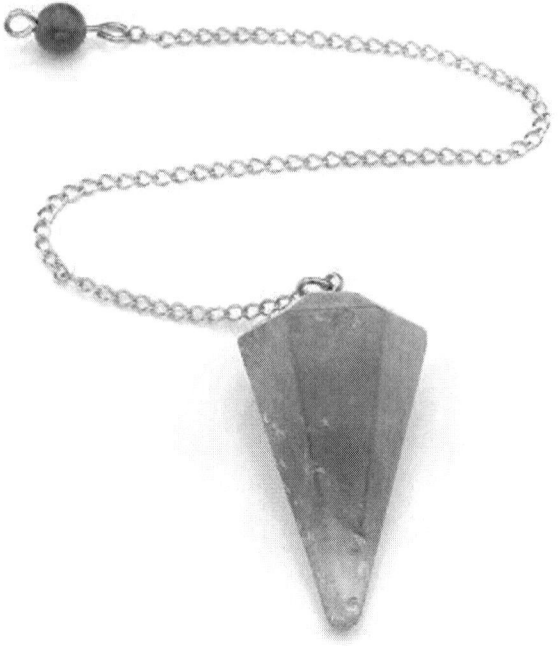

While you don't need anything to get started, there are some **things you might want to consider as you deepen your interest and commitment** to Reiki:

- Clothing – loose-fitting, comfortable clothing makes it easier, but you can also buy specific items that are recommended by the *International Association of Reiki Professionals* (*https://iarp.org*) to highlight what you do.

- A table – high quality and portable are best if you plan to practice on other people.

- A carrying case for your table.

- A timer to time your sessions.

- A comfortable swivel chair for you.

These items are better for when you have reached stage two or three, though; they aren't essential for when you're just starting out. In the beginning, you only need yourself. You could also use Reiki symbol stones, a pendulum, and cards, if you so choose.

TOP TEN REIKI
HEALING TECHNIQUES

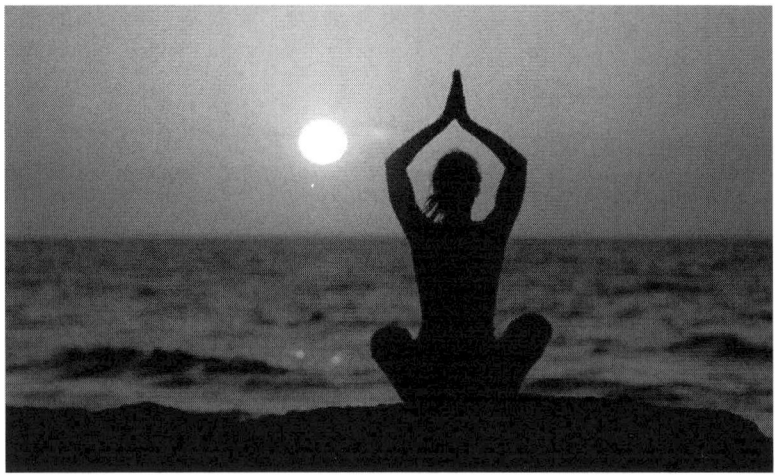

So, now that you know more about the hand positions and the basics of Reiki, it's time to look at some more techniques to enhance your healing abilities. It's best to practice your new ability as much as possible to develop your skills as far as you can.

The more you do, the more you can do.

Read on to find **ten ways you can do this**.

Intention

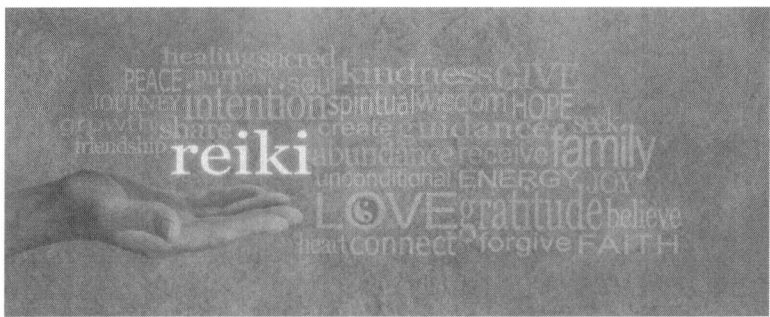

When you are Level 1 or 2, **it's important to practice on yourself every day** to hone your skills and learn more about your new magic. This will assist you in understanding your own intuition, which will guide you during your journey.

The power of intention is *very* important when it comes to Reiki. Your mind is like a magnet, so the quality of your thoughts will enhance the quality of your Reiki. You need to decide what you want to do with clarity, determination, and your full commitment, and make sure that your thoughts are positive before you begin.

Decide what you want to do and go for it. Even if self-doubt creeps up while you're performing your Reiki, just know that it's normal and not something to worry about. Don't let it derail you at all.

Try vocalizing your intention before you begin, to make sure it's at the forefront of your mind when you begin. For example: *"I intend that Reiki has charged me with enthusiasm to study well and perform well at work today."*

Just remember that the intention you begin with might not always be the result of your Reiki. Reiki works for your greater good, whatever that might be. It may not be obvious right away, but you'll soon see how you've been helped.

Mindfulness

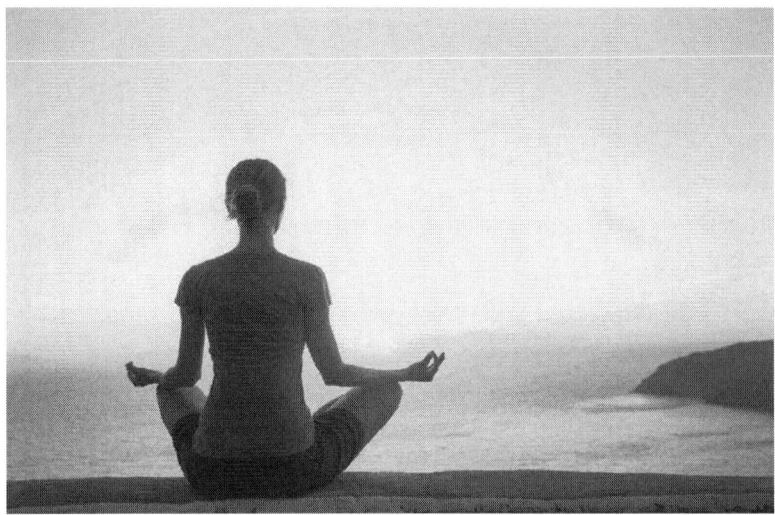

Mindfulness is a method of taking a step away from the busyness of life and being in the present moment for a period of time. That might sound simple and unnecessary, but until you start doing it, you won't realize how much time you spend worrying about the future or pondering on the past, allowing the present moment to slide past you.

Checking in with the present moment allows you to assess your mood, your body, and what's going on around you.

Professor Mark Williams, from the Oxford Mindfulness Centre, explains mindfulness clearly:

"It's easy to stop noticing the world around us. It's also easy to lose touch with the way our bodies are feeling and to end up living 'in our heads' – caught up in our thoughts without stopping to notice how those thoughts are driving our emotions and behavior.

An important part of mindfulness is reconnecting with our bodies and the sensations they experience. This means waking up to the sights, sounds, smells, and tastes of the present moment. That might be something as simple as the feel of a banister as we walk upstairs.

Another important part of mindfulness is an awareness of our thoughts and feelings as they happen moment to moment.

It's about allowing ourselves to see the present moment clearly. When we do that, it can positively change the way we see ourselves and our lives."

Mindfulness, like Reiki, is great for our well-being. Here is a list of just **some of the main benefits** as:

- Help with depression and anxiety
- Better sleep
- More energy
- Easier concentration
- No more headaches
- Higher brain function
- Better functioning immune system
- Healthier bodies

To attempt mindfulness, to see if it can help you, here is **a step-by-step guide to a breathing exercise** to get you started:

- Put yourself in a comfortable (either sitting or lying down) position and close your eyes.
- Take an exaggerated breath through your nostrils, about three seconds long.
- Exhale through your mouth, about four seconds long.
- Then breathe normally, observing the feel of your breath in your nose, your mouth, the rise and fall of your chest, the way your stomach moves.
- Focus on this for a while, but don't worry if your mind wanders. That's normal. Every time you notice it, bring your thoughts back to your breath.
- Eventually, bring your attention back into the room, and have a moment of calm with your eyes open, before you re-engage with your day.

This mindfulness exercise will assist you in applying the Five Reiki Principles to your life. It's much easier to not worry or be angry when you are concentrating on the present moment. By applying the mindfulness techniques to your everyday life and your Reiki, your actions will be more meaningful and purposeful.

Positivity

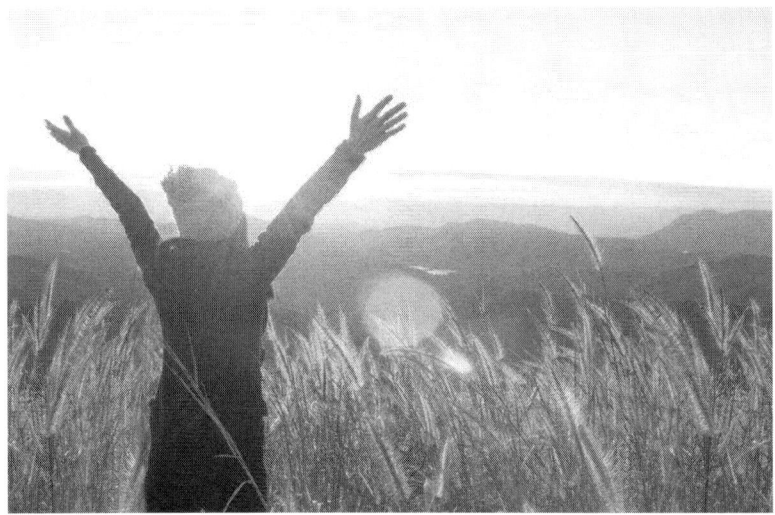

As stated before, your mind plays a massive part in your Reiki. A positive mental attitude will allow you to expand your mind and grow your talents better. Allow your mind to anticipate happiness, joy, health, and success, and the magnet of your brain will lead you in the right direction for that.

Here are some **tips to help you think more positively**:

- Recognize negative thoughts and stop them before they take root.

- Walk in nature, dance to music, play with your children – do anything that makes you happy.

- Spend time with positive people. Negativity can easily drag you down, so do your best not to get sucked up in negative, toxic relationships.

- Take care of your body. If you're healthy on the inside, you'll look good on the outside, and you'll feel much better.

- Tidy up. The clutter in your house isn't helping your mood. Get rid of it.

- Volunteer. Helping others is a good way to make you feel better.

- Get rid of stress. This might not be the easiest thing in the world. But do what you can to reduce it as much as possible. Your life will feel much better without it.

There are also some **affirmations** that can help you to get into the right mind-set. You might feel a bit silly saying them aloud at first, but that's the best way to get the full effect from them. Just think of it as you taking control of your thoughts and mind:

- I can feel amazing, just by deciding to.
- I don't need a reason to feel good.
- Knowing is not enough; we must apply. Willing is not enough; we must do.
- This too shall pass.
- In order to earn more, I must learn more.
- I control how I feel.
- I always focus on and find the good in everything.
- Life doesn't happen to me, it happens for me.
- Everything happens for a reason and a purpose, and it serves me.
- Strength doesn't come from physical capacity, it comes from an indomitable will.
- At any moment, I need to be willing to sacrifice what I am, for who I could become.
- I would rather have a mind opened by wonder than one closed by belief.

This new positive thinking of yours can assist you and your Reiki into attracting the things that you really want. Whether that's a positive life-force energy, a reenergized body and mind, or even healthier relationships, you can attract it with the power of your mind.

Unblock

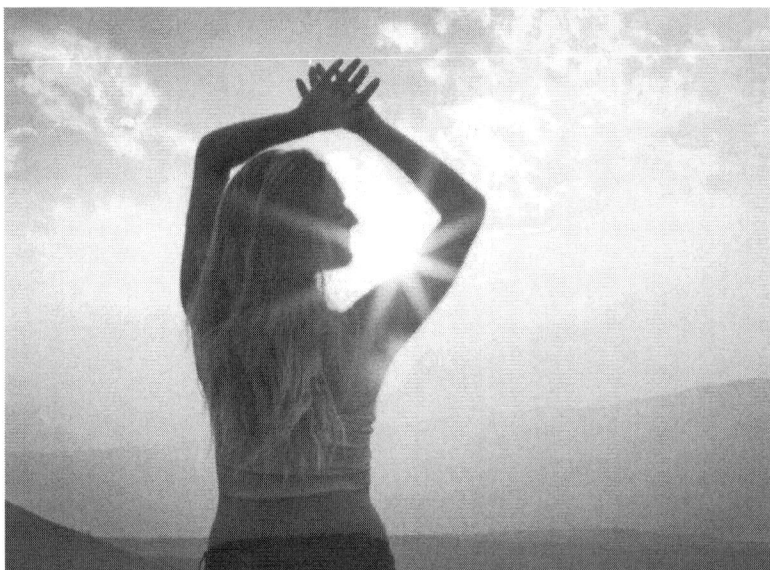

Our past does not have to define us, but it can still be there in the back of our mind, sometimes buried deep in our subconscious, affecting us in ways that we don't even realize. When you begin to experience and study Reiki, you may notice that your chakras are blocked, which may well have more to do with traumas or situations from our past that we think we've forgotten about.

These emotional blockages need to be eliminated.

Reiki can help clear these blocks in a gentle way, allowing your energy to flow a little more freely. It might take some time, but practicing every day will restore your balance and bring a sense of peace and harmony, helping you to live your life better.

Here are some **techniques to help you discover and overcome your emotional blockage**:

Identifying

- Start with a mindfulness breathing exercise to clear your mind.
- Think back over your life and any trauma that comes up. This might take a while; it may even take a few mindfulness sessions, but keep at it.
- Write it down; if more than one thing comes up, write them all down.

Releasing

- Take one memory at a time and send Reiki healing to that period in your life, that memory.

- Do this again until you feel like the memory is healed and released. Don't worry if this takes time, the effects of the trauma might be very ingrained.

Replacing

- Once you have released the memory, it's time to start thinking to the future. Visualize how you would like your life to go now that this blockage is gone.

- Send Reiki to this visualization for at least ten minutes every day.

Compassion

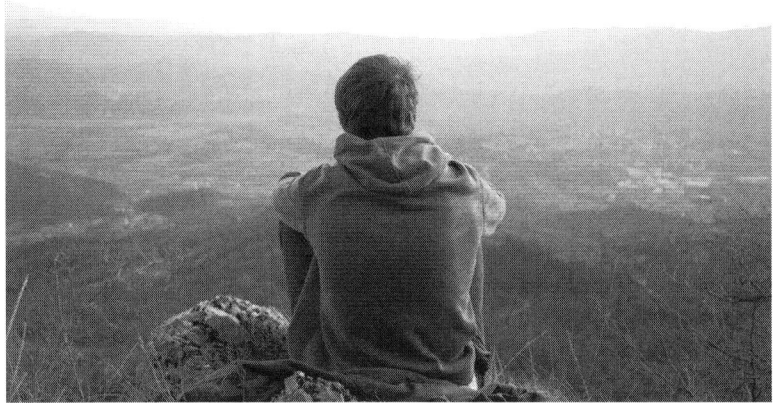

Being compassionate towards yourself and others is a simple concept that will bring you an abundance of positive results. Forgiveness, acceptance, and releasing of negativity allows everything within the body to flow more freely, in particular energy.

That's why we need to create empowering habits to ensure a happier, more fulfilled life.

Treating someone, even yourself, with Reiki is a special gift. You are given a closeness and an intimacy, which requires you to be there in the moment, fully present and with compassion. Feel deeply and understand what might be going on with the other person.

You may find that **the Reiju method helps you** with this:

- Raise hands to connect to the source of Reiki.
- Feel the energy flowing into your hands.
- Slowly lower your hands with the intention of feeling pure energy.
- Clear your mind and focus only on this energy.
- Don't move until you feel an intimate connection with the source.

Self-Treatment

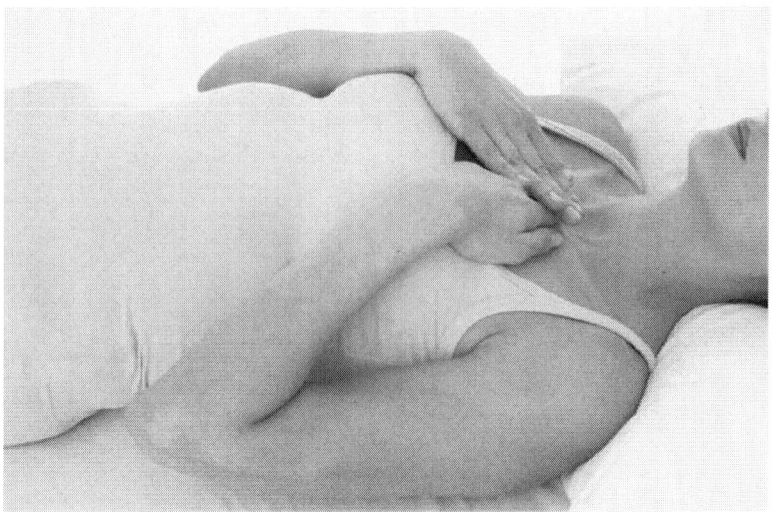

You can treat yourself with Reiki every single day, to enhance your skills and to keep your body balanced at all times. There is a simple way to do this:

Lie down in a comfortable position so you can **move your hands along your body in the following order**:

1. Crown of your head

2. Your face

3. Your throat

4. Back of your head

5. Your upper chest

6. Your lower ribs

7. Your belly button

8. Your lower abdomen

Be mindful of the present moment throughout this process, breathe steadily, and focus on the flow of Reiki. You may do it in the morning, just before opening your eyes.

This is just one example of how to practice Reiki every day. You will soon work out what works best for you as you hone your skills.

Using Your Mind

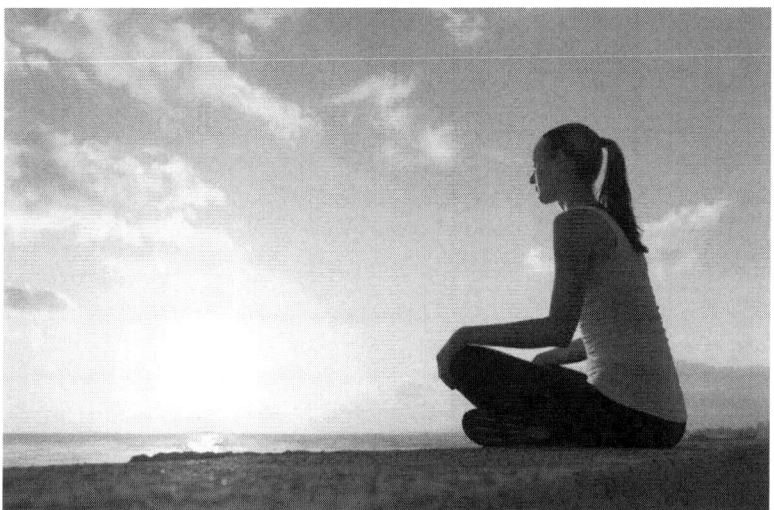

Your mind is very important in Reiki. As stated before, the intention in which you perform the Reiki makes all the difference. This can be difficult at first, and takes a lot of self-control. This is why it's good to practice on yourself every day, to hone this before you heal other people.

Here is a great **practical exercise to help you improve your concentration** and focus, which will help when healing in the future:

- Define concentration – Take your mind off multiple ideas (things) and apply it to one idea (or thing) at a time.

- Choose what you concentrate on. Often, you can take on the characteristics of what you concentrate on. For instance, some people who have been married for several years can start to resemble their spouse, and other people might start to look like their cars, pets, work projects, or hobbies.

- Observe other people while they concentrate. Go see an exciting movie, horror, action, or drama. Take a moment during the film to look at the people sitting around you. How are they acting? Typically, they sit very still, eyes will barely blink, and their breathing has slowed. Only a major distraction could interrupt this stream of attention. Make note of these physical signs to guide yourself with ways to enhance how you concentrate.

- Apply your full concentration on what you are doing and avoid multitasking, or attempting to perform more than one activity at a time. Avoiding distractions by working in a quiet place helps, as well. Filter out constant noise and visual stimulation (for example, TV and devices), which always make concentrating more difficult.

- Learn to remain calm. Calm, focused energy can result in deep concentration by directing or increasing your life force. The more conscious, cosmic energy you control, the better. When your energy is scattered, it isn't functional.

- Use techniques to control and increase your energy. Energization Exercises from *Paramahansa Yogananda*, for example, can help you take that important first step in controlling your energy and concentrating deeply.

- Make time for breaks in your schedule. On these breaks, you could go outside to take a brisk walk or just breathe deeply. Do this frequently, and you can feel recharged and ready to focus with more creativity on your project.

- Meditate; this is the most powerful technique to enhance concentration. Practice a couple simple techniques for at least five minutes per day.

- Observe your breathing as you meditate. Don't try to control it. This can help you learn how to focus on one thing at a time. As you observe, your breathing will slow down. Then, your mind will follow along, which has been well-documented scientifically. This moves you into a peaceful, yet dynamic, state. This makes you feel recharged and your mind receptive to creativity.

The more you do this, the more centered you will become. This will not only help with Reiki, but calming the mind all the time, stopping your brain from being so busy, and focusing only on the present moment.

Healing Relationships

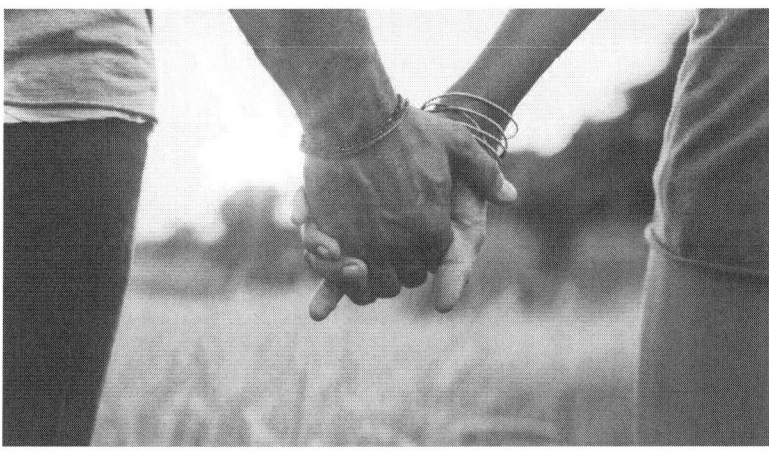

Relationships can get fractured through life. Sometimes, through our own fault; sometimes, through the faults of others; sometimes, it just happens. This can leave sadness and empty holes in our lives that we wish to repair. Whether this relates to romantic relationships, family bonds, or friendships, Reiki can help you.

The first step is to recognize that relationships are a living organism with their own energy. Once you see it like this, it's easier to detach a little, to focus your healing energy. It's also easier to see why this might have gone wrong, where the imbalance has come from, so it becomes easier to repair.

Reiki always works for the greater good, so it can assist in healing negativity, improving communication, better understanding – but if it doesn't work, it might be worth working out why. Perhaps the relationship cannot be healed for a good reason and it's time to leave it alone.

This comes with Level 2 of Attunement, once you can start healing other people. That's when you can **try out some practical exercises**, such as this one:

- *Recognize* – who is the relationship with? Why has it fallen apart? Writing this down might be helpful.

- *Intent* – why is this relationship worth saving? What does it mean to you? How will your life improve if you take them back?

- *Concentrate* – focus on your intention. Make sure you aren't being selfish. Work out what comes next. **Use this in the following exercise**:
    1. Use a picture of the person you shared the broken relationship with.

2. Calmly breathe in and out to invoke Universal Energy, which will pass through your palms as you hold the picture.

3. As you exhale, visualize the energy in your breath coursing through your bloodstream to your fingers.

4. The person might appear to be imbued with red, yellow, blue, or green light.

5. Speak your acknowledgement of this relationship, its importance, aloud in order to invoke this energy.

6. Speak that acknowledgement about 3 to 6 times to establish the energy.

7. Speak your intentions aloud about 3 to 6 times to infuse them with energy.

8. Slowly inhale, then exhale completely, as you prepare to heal this relationship by sending out this energy.

9. Aim your hands and direct the energy toward the picture.

10. Be thankful for Universal Energy and that person as you complete this exercise.

Reenergizing

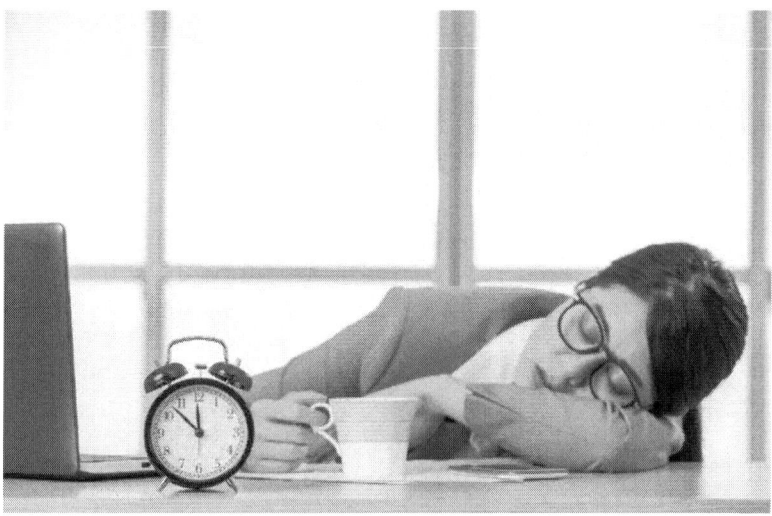

It's so easy to get bogged down in the race of life. Everything seems to move at breakneck speed, and it's hard to keep your energy levels high. Reiki is wonderful for removing the negative energy from your body and replacing it with positive, which will help uplift you. It is also wonderful for resting your mind, calming the busy thoughts that will have a negative effect on your body, and leaving you rested. This will, of course, bring your energy levels up.

Here is a great **exercise to help reenergize your body and mind**, to recharge and leave you feeling more like yourself:

- Inhale deeply through your mouth, then exhale slowly through your nose.

- Visualize a ball, golden and glowing, floating above your head. Visualize it floating down, then joining the violet head chakra. The violet, gold rays are spreading to your body's systems, which will energize the eyes and nervous system.

- Repeat, "I am at peace and divinely guided and protected," to yourself.

- Next, visualize the glowing ball separating gently from the violet chakra so it can move down and merge with the third eye chakra. Picture it blending with the third eye's indigo wheel. Now these indigo, gold rays can energize the eyes and ears, nose, pituitary gland, and hypothalamus. While you imagine this, repeat, "I follow my instincts and am open to new people, situations, and ideas," to yourself.

- Watch the glowing ball slowly separate from the third eye chakra and descend into the throat chakra's blue wheel. Visualize the blue, gold rays as they energize the bronchial, throat, upper lungs, upper stomach, and digestive tract areas. Repeat, "I trust, respect, and love my creativity and feel safe in expressing my feelings," to yourself.

- Next, see the glowing ball separate from the throat chakra and float down to the heart chakra's green wheel. Watch the green, gold rays energize the arms, heart and blood, thymus, upper liver, and lower lungs. Say, "Love is everywhere and is my life's purpose," to yourself.

- From there, watch the glowing ball separate from the heart chakra and blend with the yellow wheel of the solar plexus chakra. These yellow, gold rays will spread to the spleen, liver, pancreas, intestines and digestive system, and gall bladder. Say, "I am worthy to receive the best of life and trust that worthiness," to yourself.

- Next, visualize the glowing ball separating from the solar plexus chakra to join with the orange wheel of the sacral chakra. Picture the orange, gold rays energizing your whole reproductive system. Repeat, "What I have and what do is enough," to yourself.

- Then, imagine the glowing ball separating from the sacral chakra and joining with the red wheel of the base chakra. Watch as the red, gold rays spread throughout the excretory system and energize the lower limbs, kidneys and bladder, and spine. Say, "I love my legs, how they support me. I love my feet, how they guide me. I am always secure and safe," to yourself.

- Keep inhaling through your mouth, exhaling through your nose. Feel all your disruptive emotions flying away; feel the abundance of love flowing. You are totally at peace, calm. Feel fully relaxed and grounded.

- Visualize only light surrounding you. Your aura is expanding, protected by white light. You are now protected, where no negative energy can reach you.

- Reiki has now fully energized you. Picture you standing in front of yourself, then pass yourself Reiki. You are healing yourself, family; forgiving yourself, family.

- Use Reiki to energize the 5 elements. Visualize each of the elements in your hands to thank, energize, and bless them with Reiki. Imagine that you are holding earth, water, fire, air, then space/cosmos in your hands, then watch the Reiki energy flow through each element.

- This is the end of your meditation. Progress out of the meditation slowly, stretching your arms and legs and returning from your head, ears, torso, then your legs from the very tips of your toes. Open your eyes slowly to regain awareness of your environment. Now you are fully charged and ready to face your environment.

Attracting Abundance

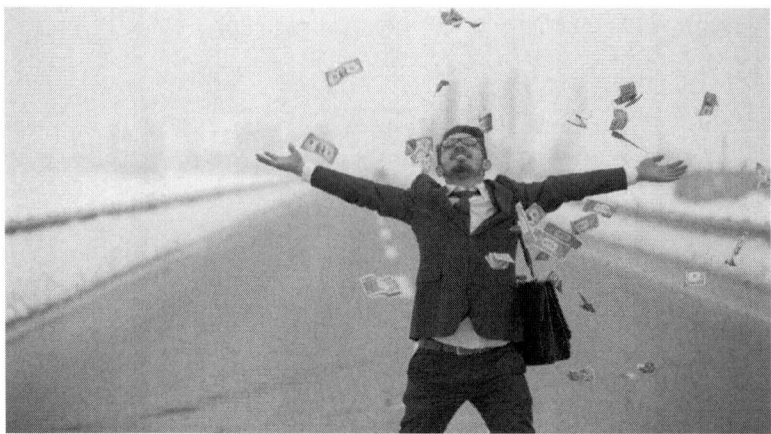

Attracting success and other things in abundance, whether that be success, money, or something else, Reiki can help you with it. Sometimes, the thing holding you back could be an emotional blockage that you don't even realize is there, stopping you from getting where you want to be.

Here are some **techniques to help** with this:

- Use Reiki to create a list of things that could enhance your quality of life, supporting the highest good.

- With each of the items on that list, you will want to make a heart-mind connection by invoking Reiki's distant and mental/emotional symbols. Consider your feelings as you think of them. What energetic essence does each item hold, and how will they add to your quality of life?

- Consider entering a 21-day Reiki process to draw the listed items into your life. Employ the distant, power, and mental/emotional symbols each day by invoking their names, drawing them, or visualizing them.

- After you call the energy of the symbols, hold that list in your hands to pass Reiki energy directly into it. Now, verbally express gratitude for the good things in your life.

- Allow Reiki energy to flow until it feels complete, stops, or merely slows. Be sure to close this session with prayer.

FIVE POWERFUL
GUIDED MEDITATIONS

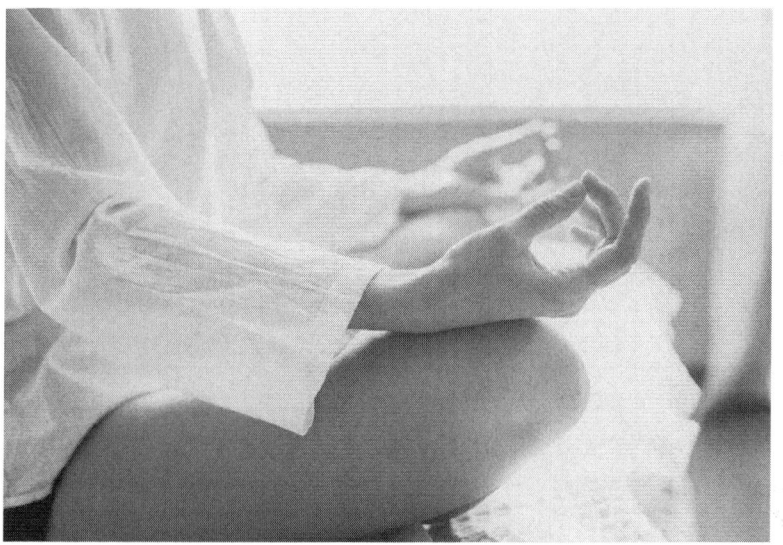

There are lots of excellent guided meditations to help you with your Reiki. Getting in touch with your inner self is the best way to explore your connection to your Reiki energy and your chakras as well. There are many resources for this that can be easily found, but here are **five guided meditations** to get you started.

Chakra Meditation

Chakra meditation uses Reiki energy to clear blockages and to promote the healing flow of energy throughout your body. Just like with Reiki, the intention while performing this mediation is vital to the outcome.

- Start by sitting in a comfortable position, keeping your spine straight – comfortably, not rigid. Then focus on each part of your body, working up from your feet. Relax each part of your body, allowing any stress to melt away.

- Next, focus on your breathing. Let your breathing become deep and even. Gently bring back your mind if it wanders. You want to maintain focus on each breath you take. Picture oxygen entering your lungs, then passing into your bloodstream. It's nourishing the cells, muscles, and organs in your body. Each breath is removing toxins from your body.

- Third, picture your heart beating, the body functioning perfectly. Visualize how the parts function in harmony, how your breath sustains the whole body and each of these parts. Meditate on how your breath is a life-giving force for your entire body.

- Fourth, visualize that you are breathing in a life-giving energy along with the oxygen. This energy will manifest with a yellow-orange color. Visualize the energy infusing your aura and encompassing your entire body. Picture your aura growing brighter, stronger, as it charges with energy. Allow the aura to grow brighter gradually, keeping the energy flowing with every breath.

- Fifth, energize the individual chakras. Begin with the root chakra and imagine a clockwise movement of energy. As you breathe in, more energy propels this movement and keeps it bright and strong. Then, imagine more of that life-giving energy coming up out of the earth, adding to the moving energy seated in the root chakra.

- Sixth, move up through the remaining chakras: sacral, solar plexus, heart, throat, head, and then, the crown. Infuse each one with that life-giving energy. Proceed slowly and spend more time with one chakra if needed. This process works better if you start from the bottom, flow up, and do not skip a chakra. One chakra influences the chakra that follows it. Energizing chakras from high to low may produce adverse effects.

- Finally, visualize the chakras simultaneously being boosted by the energy coming from your breath and the earth. Focus on your chakras and aura growing clearer, brighter, being supercharged by the life-giving energy.

- Now you can open your eyes. Take a couple of minutes to relax with your eyes open. Focus on your body and how energized you feel. Give yourself 15-30 minutes to practice in each sitting.

Third Eye Opening

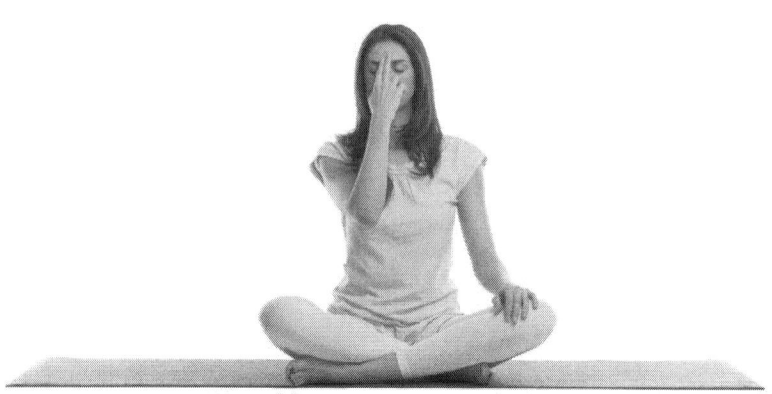

Your third eye is the 'eye of insight.' It offers you much clearer vision and an examination of the world around you. It's extremely important to see your Reiki energy as clearly as you need to. Keeping your third eye balanced keeps your body energy flowing too.

Third eye opening uses Reiki energy to clear your mind and calm your thoughts, reenergizing you and bringing you back to a place of peace. It will also assist you in following the Reiki Principles better because you'll be able to see things clearer, with less of an emotional attachment clouding your judgement.

- Plan to take 30 minutes for meditation.
- Eliminate distractions, especially, by turning off your phone.
- Wear comfortable clothes.
- Align your chakras by sitting in the lotus position. You can lie down if the lotus position isn't comfortable.
- Relax your body muscles, start with your feet and work your way up.
- Move to a breathing meditation and visualize each part of your body relaxing.
- Imagine a wave of calm washing over your entire body. It rises through your body, generating warmth.
- Draw this energy between your eyebrows, right into the center of your head.

- Let go of attachments, any singular thought; clear your mind of running thoughts, as if nothing matters at all.

- Your body becomes lighter, feel gravity disappear.

- Focus on your breath, then imagine a white ball of light rotating 360 degrees at the center of your mind. Watch this ball expand, accept its presence. Welcome it into your possession.

- As the ball expands, allow its light to stream out from your forehead.

- Let your thoughts rise and fall naturally.

- Welcome the light in, stay open to acknowledging what is presented to you, such as information, pictures, or colors.

- This is the time to connect, seeking a spirit guide, God, or Mother Nature. You can call out with your voice or silently inside your head.

- Speak this calling as you would a mantra. Do so until you recognize a response.

- Practice caution when you recognize the response. Sudden movements or shock can interrupt your meditation.

- At this point, you could ask your third eye for information, insight, or a message. Otherwise, you could just be in the present and take whatever comes from such an enlightening moment.

- This may seem dream-like, but with regular practice, the experiences will become familiar. You'll eventually learn how to manifest and cultivate higher knowledge within your physical being.

Reiki New Moon Meditation

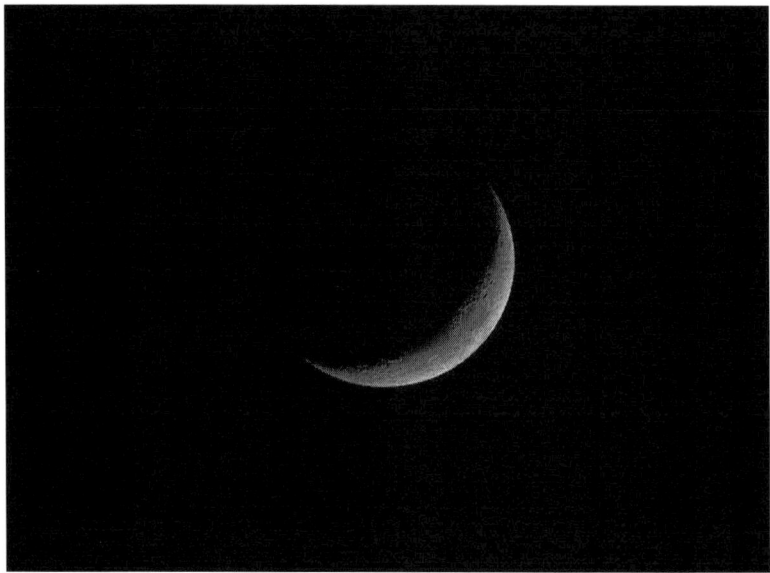

For Reiki healing, energy from the moon plays a very important role. The lunar cycle dispels energies toward certain goals and intentions, and a new moon is the best for new beginnings. When you want to establish a new path or start thriving, **this mediation is useful to invoke the right energy.**

- Start with a prayer of thanks that you can be an open channel where Reiki can flow; additionally, ask to keep your ego and personality in check, so Reiki can flow in the truest, clearest form. Express gratitude for being open to receive guidance from any masters or angels who provide assistance.

- Draw an Usui power symbol to prepare your energy field. This will strengthen your light and help move energy into your auric field. Draw smaller versions of the Usui power symbols over each chakra, starting with the base chakra. Pause here to move Reiki toward the solar plexus and heart chakras.

- Pray to the ascended spiritual beings and masters, the Divine. Warmly welcome these beings, and grant them admission to help you determine your sacred intention and manifest those intentions. Give thanks for their presence.

- Put your sacred intention for this meditation, even your intention for world service, down on paper. You might even draw a symbol that clarifies your vision. Include your personal goals, and you should employ the Usui mental/emotional symbol. Using a new moon journal, for example, would be an appropriate channel for these notes. State your written intention, then channel the Reiki mental/emotional energy there.

- Visualize building a bridge of light between the spiritual masters' hearts and yours by employing the Usui distant healing symbol. Feel your soul connecting to these souls; watch the appearance of separation disappear. Recognize the oneness of creation, then remember Reiki is not confined by space or time. Note: if you are attuned to the Reiki Master or Karuna Reiki® symbols you can add them to the meditation.

- Take as much as needed to meditate, then transmit Reiki energy.

- Offer another prayer filled with gratitude.

- Declare the intention of disconnecting from the meditation by drawing a large power symbol over your body. Recognize that each spiritual master is also disconnecting, then allow yourself to return to your individual life expression aligned with your soul's purpose and with clarity.

Healing Meditation

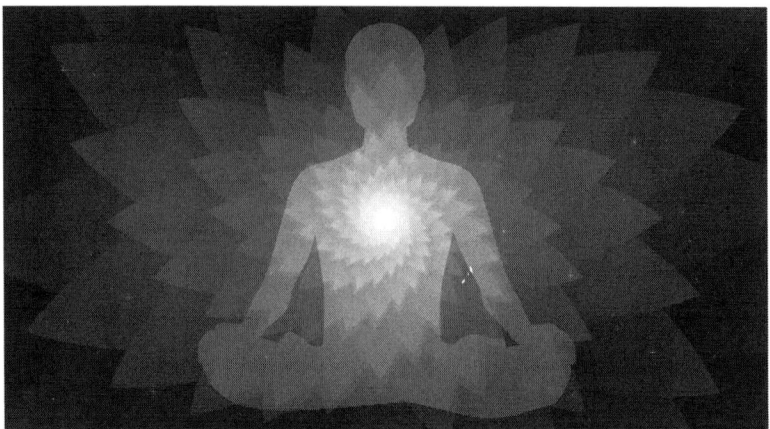

Healing energy is needed to clear emotional blockages and to reenergize yourself. **This mediation works with the universe's energy and your chakras** to ensure that the energy flowing through your body is unbroken.

- Close your eyes gently, and focus on your breathing, your body; relax your belly, clear your mind.

- Connect with the ground, feel its support, below.

- Let the sounds around you simply be there.

- Take notice of the light, the shadows, the air touching your skin.

- Visualize the sky, its horizons stretching around the globe, the earth carrying you.

- Clear your mind of thoughts, feelings it no longer needs. Cleanse your body of energies it no longer needs.

- Draw your energy back to your core by grounding yourself in the moment.

- Allow yourself to sense the space around you. Breathe intentionally, heighten your awareness of its entering and leaving your body, the sound and temperature.

- Breathe into your root chakra, taking the nourishment of life-force energy into your chakra of belonging.

- Visualize your root chakra connecting to the earth. Picture red, the color of the earth, and infuse your base chakra with it. Focus on the present; let it ground you, empower you; embody this moment. Allow your chakra to take the energy it needs. Repeat, "I have every right to be here"; "Earth supports me"; "I am here, as I am," to yourself.

- Move your awareness up to your sacral chakra, the hara, of pleasure, emotional intelligence, movement, choice, and creativity.

- Breathe into your sacral chakra, taking the nourishment of life-force energy into your hara. Picture the color orange, the color of a warm sunset, and infuse your second chakra with it. Allow your hara to be filled. Find balance; be empowered and motivated. Repeat, "I am nourished"; "I allow myself to honor my needs," to yourself.

- Move your awareness up to your solar plexus. The personal power chakra.

- Breathe into your solar plexus chakra, taking the nourishment of life-force energy into your power chakra. Picture yellow, the color of sun beams, and infuse your third chakra with them. You will feel nurtured, restored, and replenished. Allow your power chakra to take the energy it needs. Repeat, "I value myself"; "I am enough"; "I am worthy of gold," to yourself.

- Move your awareness up to your heart chakra. The unconditional love and self-development chakra.

- Breathe into your heart chakra, taking the nourishment of life-force energy into your unconditional love chakra. Picture green, the color of renewal or spring, and infuse your fourth chakra with it. You will experience healing and being nourished. Allow your love chakra to take the energy it needs. Repeat, "I am nourished by love"; "I will freely give and receive love," to yourself.

- Move your awareness up to your throat chakra. The willpower and self-expression chakra.

- Breathe into your throat chakra, taking nourishment of life-force energy into your willpower chakra. Picture blue, the color of the sky, and infuse your fifth chakra with it. You will sense a freedom of creativity and self-expression, an opening or clearing, and losing the desire for control. Allow your willpower chakra to take the energy it needs. Repeat, "I will follow life's flow"; "I speak, hear my truth"; "I freely express myself" to yourself.

- Move your awareness up to your third eye chakra, the intuition and wisdom chakra. Breathe into your third eye chakra, taking nourishment of life-force energy into your intuition chakra.

- Picture indigo, the color of the night sky, and infuse your sixth chakra with it. You will be balanced and soothed and experience understanding, clarity, and insight. Allow your intuition chakra to take the energy it needs. Repeat, "Everything happens as it should," to yourself.

- Move your awareness up to your crown chakra, the oneness chakra. Breathe into your crown chakra, taking nourishment of life-force energy into your oneness chakra.

- Picture the color light violet and infuse your seventh chakra with it. You will feel harmony, restored, and balanced. Allow your oneness chakra to take the energy it needs. Repeat, "I become as one with the Whole, with the Universe," to yourself.

- In your own time, come back to your whole self, back to the movement of your breathing, back to your core. Breathe into your center. Repeat, "I am whole just as I am"; "I am enough," to yourself. Let the energy of these words infuse your emotions, mind, body, and, spirit. Take all the energy that you need.

- Raise your awareness to the air touching your skin and to the sounds surrounding you.

- Slowly close your chakras down, making the clear intention can be enough. Focus on the support of the earth below you. Become aware of your feelings. Remember the unique, beautiful soul that you are, holding yourself with unconditional loving kindness.

- In your own time, close this meditation.

Reiki Calm Meditation

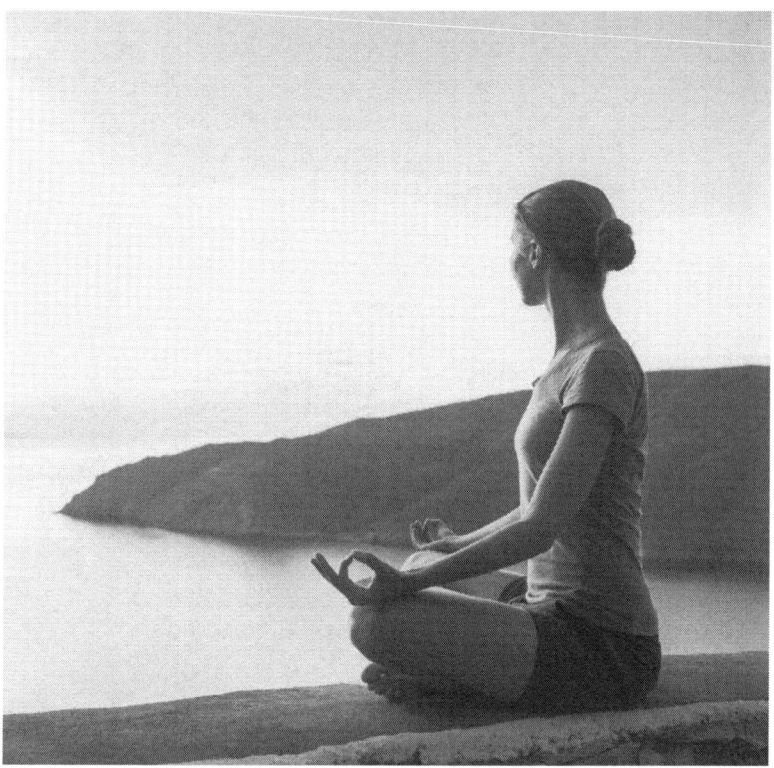

A sense of calm and peace is essential for everyone. Life is so busy and chaotic, full of stressful thoughts and pressures, which stops the energy flowing through your body properly. This can have a direct effect on all areas of your life, so **taking a moment to find calm is very useful**.

- Slowly inhale at the count of four and release the breath through the mouth. Do it one more time and relax.

- Count from 5 to 1, your body will start releasing all the ache and tension stored in the muscles and drift into a deeply calm and serene state.

    - 5…Your toes, feet, calf and knee muscles are loose and limber now.

    - 4…Your thigh, pelvis, and lower back muscles are relaxed now.

    - 3…Your hands, shoulders, abdominal and chest muscles are relaxed now.

    - 2…Your upper back, neck, and facial muscles are loose now.

– 1…Your scalp muscles and hair follicles are relaxed now.

- Now visualize yourself walking on a seashore at the time of sunrise. The fresh cool air you are breathing on the shore is immensely refreshing and rejuvenating. As you walk along this beautiful shore, you find a comfortable place to sit down. You gaze around and see Divine Sun slowly making his way through the blanket of clouds to welcome you and the world. The sun is your guard and protector throughout your meditation and presence on the shore.

- (Do the exercise of chakra healing below for as much time as you want to heal each chakra, like 4-5 min or more, and then move to the next chakra.)

- The Reiki energy of the highest dimension is now flowing through your root chakra to heal, align, and balance it. Visualize that waves filled with the color red are gushing towards the shore, cleansing your root chakra from inside out.

- (Follow the instruction above for each chakra: sacral, solar plexus, heart, throat, third eye, and crown.)

- Visualize roots coming out of your feet and going 10-15 feet deep into Mother Earth. Reiki energy now flows through your root chakra, sending all the excess and pent-up energy from your body into Mother Earth to ground your energy field.

- Thank Masters of Reiki Energy, Guardian Angels, Archangel Michael, and Divine Sun for healing. Visualize yourself in a protective ball of blue light.

As previously stated, there are many resources for guided meditations to help get you started. For further reading, check out *Chakras* website at _chakras.info/opening-third-eye._

SIGNIFICANCE OF
REIKI SYMBOLS

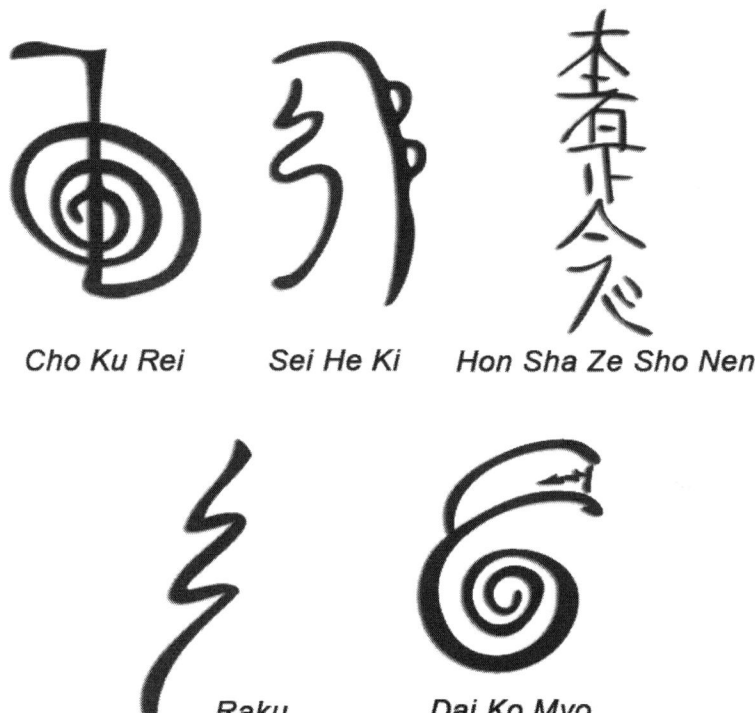

Cho Ku Rei   Sei He Ki   Hon Sha Ze Sho Nen

Raku   Dai Ko Myo

There are five Reiki symbols that you might like to learn on your new journey into this new power. They do not hold any special power themselves, other than that of empowerment. The symbols are sacred and refer to the Japanese name or intention. While you might not need them, a lot of people find it extremely useful to know and use these.

The symbols are significant because Dr. Usui received the symbols in his mystical experience on Mount Kurama as he was developing Reiki. They are Japanese and were around before this time, having been used in Buddhism, but this attachment from the founder gives users a stronger bond to him.

They are used by drawing them with your finger into the air, while stating your intention to hone your power and make it that much more powerful.

Cho Ku Rei

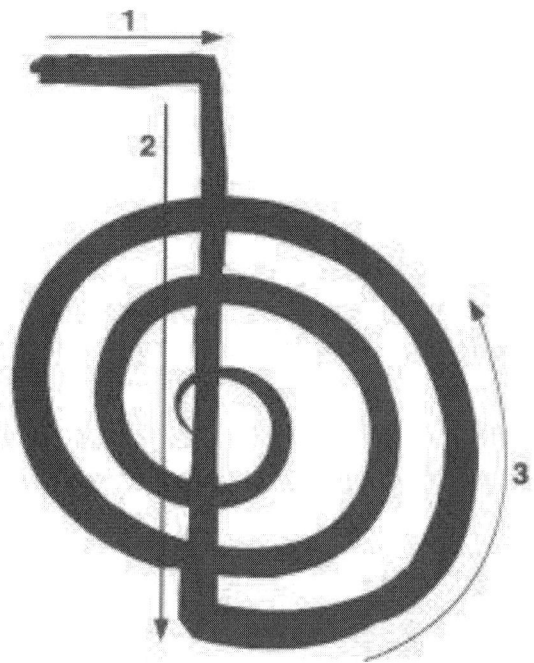

This is the *power* symbol and can be used to increase or decrease power depending on which way it's drawn. It's performed with the intention of 'turning the light switch on,' and is best used before or after a session. The coil is the important part because it expands or decreases your energy depending on what you want.

Sei He Ki

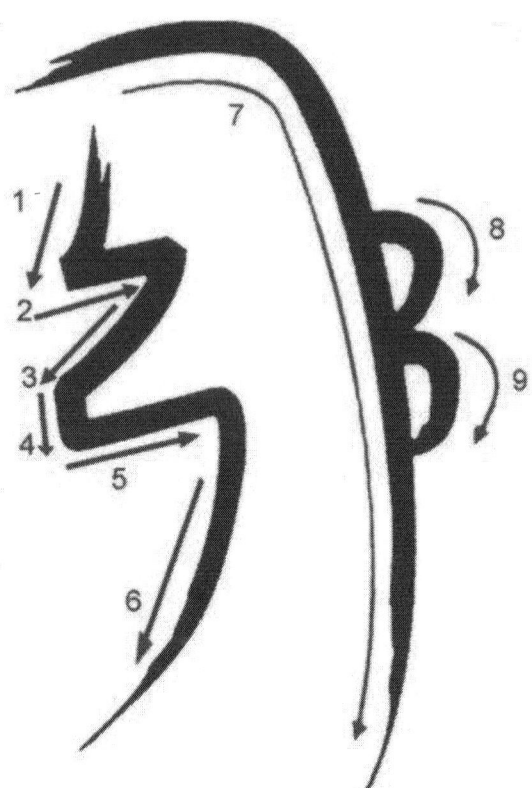

This is the *harmony* symbol, performed with the intention of balance. It purifies and is used for mental and emotional well-being. The symbol is drawn with a sweeping gesture to rid the body of anything negative or toxic at the beginning of a session. This includes past trauma.

Hon Sha Ze Sho Nen

HON-SHA-ZE-SHO-NEN

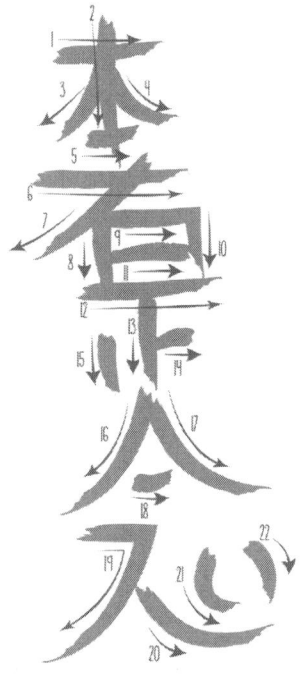

This is the *distance* symbol and can be used to help send Reiki over a distance. It's sent with the intention of timelessness. It isn't sent with a specific purpose; it's merely to bring a closeness and connection, performed at the end of a session.

Dai Ko Myo (or Da Koo Mo)

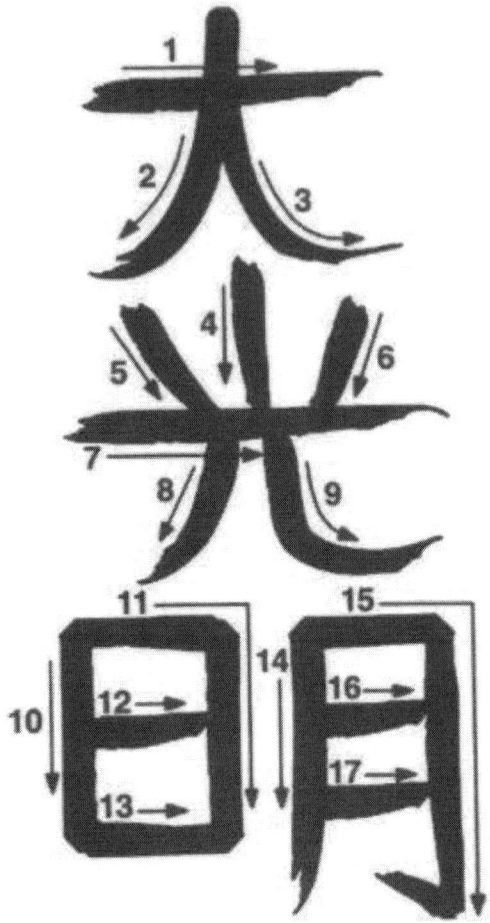

This is the *master* symbol and is performed with the intention of enlightenment. This combines the first three symbols and is used to enhance the healing effects of any Reiki. It's the most complex to draw but very powerful, done at the beginning of a session.

Da Koo Moo is another version called *Tibetan Dai Ko Mio* or *Dai Ko Myo Contemporary Master Symbol*. This symbol is quite beautiful and powerful – it is quite efficiently used in Karuna Reiki - but has nothing to do with Traditional Reiki according to Mikao Usui.

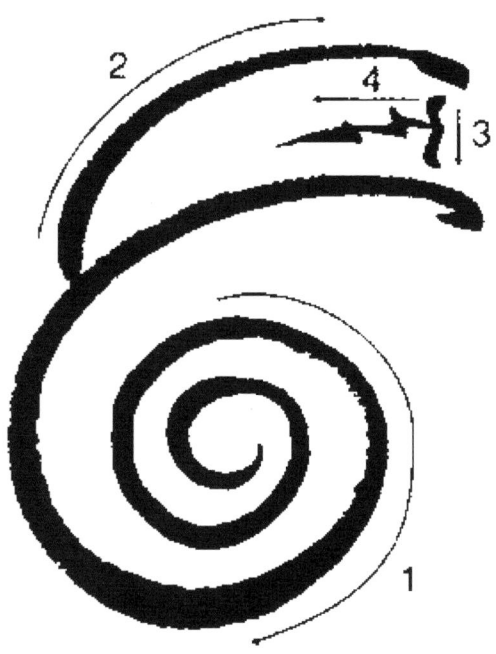

Raku

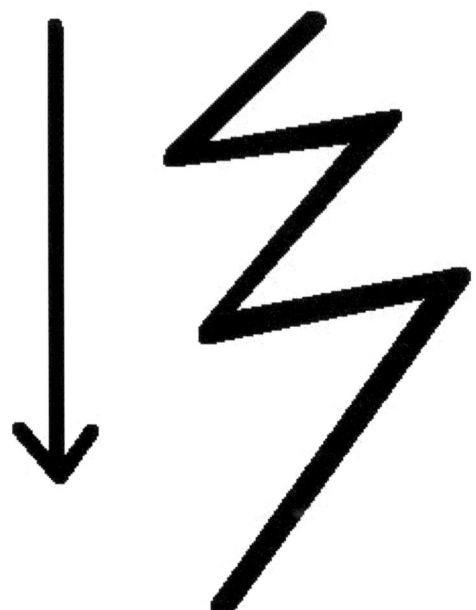

This is the *completion* symbol, and it's performed by Reiki Masters with the intention of grounding. This seals the healing in all the seven chakras and enhances and awakens energies, done at the end of a session.

These symbols can be used as you need them and don't have to be used alone. You can use them together for more benefit.

Here are some **extra uses for the symbols** so you can get the best out of them:

- *Cho Ku Rei* can also be drawn over doors and entrances to provide protection.
- *Cho Ku Rei* is also good for protecting food and ridding it of the negative energies it might have picked up on its way to you.
- *Sei He Ki* is great for enhancing your affirmations.
- *Sei He Ki* is also wonderful for helping you to memorize information.
- *Cho Ku Rei* and *Sei He Ki* can help get rid of a bad habit.

- *Cho Ku Rei, Sei He Ki, Hon Sha Ze Sho Nen,* and *Cho Ku Rei* repeated after one another will send Reiki to a sick child.

- Use *Cho Ku Rei, Sei He Ki, Hon Sha Ze Sho Nen,* and *Cho Ku Rei* to send Reiki to a future event.

GLOSSARY

There are some terms that you might come across while learning Reiki, and you'll need to know what they mean, so **here are the most important terms:**

A

Advanced Reiki Training (ART)	A student achieves Level 3, or 'Master' level, attunement, but has not been instructed in passing attunements to others. Also known as Master-Practitioner Level or Level 3a. For Usui/Tibetan Reiki training, the common Level 3 gets broken down to two parts. ART includes 'non-traditional' concepts – meditation on Reiki symbols, Reiki guide meditations, Reiki crystal grids, healing attunements, Antahkarana symbol, and psychic surgery – and emphasizes 'personal mastery.'
Ai-Reiki	Being in harmony with Reiki.
American Reiki Association, Inc.	Founded by Takata-Sensei and Barbara Ray in 1980. Is now operating as the RTIA (the Radiance Technique International Association, Inc.).
Anshin Ritsumei	State where a person's mind is at peace, and one's life's purpose can be perceived. (Alternately: *Dai-anjin*)
Antahkarana	A cube with 'L' shapes on each surface. This 'non-traditional' Reiki symbol is claimed to have a Tibetan origin, but this has not been validated. It is also said the Antahkarana is a remedy for any ailment.
Aoki, Huminori (or Fuminori)	Chairman of the Nagoya Reiki Lab, teaches *Reido* Reiki – his unique system that combines elements of Japanese and Western traditions. Wrote the book, *The Reiki Healing*.

| Attunement (also: Initiation or Empowerment) | (In Japanese: *Denju*) Each Level or Degree focuses on this sacred process, which is administered by a Reiki Master or Teacher. A student's energy centers and etheric field are essentially recalibrated or re-patterned. This enables a student to interact with Reiki energy. |

B

Beaming	Non-contact method of Reiki treatment where a Practitioner stands within line of sight of the client and projects (or 'beams') Reiki energy. This is different from distant treatment because the client is present for treatment.
'Blue Book'	Written by Takata-Sensei's granddaughter (Phyllis Lei Furumoto) and Paul Mitchell (from the Reiki Alliance) in 1985. Includes historical data presented by Hawayo Takata, information about the Reiki Alliance, Takata-Sensei's diary excerpts, and pictures of Takata-Sensei and Phyllis Lei Furumoto, Usui-Sensei, and Hayashi-Sensei.
Blue Kidney Breath	Cross-reference: Breath of the Fire Dragon.
Breath of the Fire Dragon	Unique breathing technique employed in *Raku Kei* Reiki. Known by various names, but two well-known names are Violet Breath (*Tera Mai*) and 'Blue Kidney Breath.'
Byogen Chiryo-Ho	Technique comparable to *Genetsu-ho*, whose name translates to: 'Treating the origin of a disease.' *Byo* = disease; *Gen* = origin; *Chiryo* = treatment
Byosen Reikan-Ho	Reiki technique where a Practitioner sends their hands through a client's energy field (or aura) to determine energetic fluctuations. Specifically, an 'energetic sensation' in areas of dis-ease or dis-harmony. This is called 'Scanning' in Western traditions.
	Byosen is also concerned with inspiration or intuition. 'Reikan' in the full name has been translated as 'inspiration.' However, in a more accurate sense, this term refers to 'spiritual intuition' or what we could describe as 'psychic sensitivity.' (Alternatively: *Byosen*)

C

Chakra Kassei Kokyu-Ho	Breathing method from *Gendai Reiki-ho* that activates the chakras.
Choku Rei (Cho-ku-rei)	First Usui Reiki symbol out of four. Referred to as the 'power' symbol within Reiki from the Takata lineage (*Usui Shiki Ryoho*). This symbol is also known as the 'focus' symbol in other Japanese lineages. *Choku Rei* was translated by Takata-Sensei to mean 'put the [spiritual] power here.' However, it can also be translated to: 'Direct Spirit' or 'in the presence of the Spirit(s).'
Chuden	Reiki level of training that falls between *Shoden* and *Okuden*. *Chu* = middle or second; *Den* = teaching
Chu Tanden (see: Tanden)	Energy center situated deep inside a person's chest.
Crystal Grid	Crystals charged with Reiki energy that appear within a specific geometrical layout. They are designed to emit protective or therapeutic influence continually.

D

Dai Ko Myo	Name for the last three Usui Reiki symbols. This is often referred to as the 'master' symbol within Reiki from the Takata lineage (*Usui Shiki Ryoho*).
	The three words *Dai*, *Ko*, and *Myo*, written in *kanji* actually constitute the 'symbol.' This name literally translates to: 'Great shining light.' Making reference to the Light of Wisdom, how illumination "dawns on us" and the 'Enlightened Nature,' 'Radiant Light of Wisdom,' or a deity's (e.g., Vidyaraja, Buddha, or Bodhisattva) radiance.
Dai Shihan (see: Shihan)	Reiki (in some Japanese styles) level above *Shihan* (meaning: master/teacher). For those styles, one achieves the *Dai Shihan* level in order to initiate students to *Shihan* level.
	Dai Shihan has been translated to mean 'Grand Master.'
Dashu-Ho	Cross-reference: *Uchite Chiryo-Ho*.
Den	Term found in titles of Levels or grades used within most Japanese Reiki traditions, such as *Shoden*, *Okuden*, *Shinpiden*. *Den* = teachings

Denju	Western Reiki process of attunement employed by Takata-Sensei. *Denju* refers to the fullest meaning of 'initiation,' which consists of energetic 'attunement' and the teachings that go with it.
Dento Reiki (-Ryoho)	Term often used to indicate *Usui Reiki Ryoho* or 'traditional Reiki.'
Distant Attunement	Non-traditional practice of projecting Reiki energy on a student or client who is not physically present to receive attunement treatment. Most Japanese Reiki traditions (for example, *Hekikuu*, *Gendai*, or *Komyo*) do not allow this practice (distant *reiju* or attunements [*denju*]).

The founder of *Hekikuu* Reiki, Kenji Hamamoto, says:

"To effectively assist the student to awaken to Reiki, the teacher needs to be present, needs to be able to watch for the physiological signs that the process is actually unfolding; to receive tangible energetic feedback. It would be disrespectful to the student to merely raise the hands at a distance, take their money, and hope."

Distant (also: Remote) Treatment	Performing Reiki treatment for a client who cannot be physically present.
Distant Symbol	Cross-reference: *Hon Sha Ze Sho Nen*.
Do	'Path' or 'Way' with a spiritual or philosophical nature.
Dojo	Term that refers to a space for pursuing meditation and spiritual discipline. Commonly refers to a training hall for martial arts today. *Dojo* = The Place of the Way
Dumo	Used within *Raku Kei* Reiki along with other modern Reiki traditions. *Dumo* = Tibetan master symbol

E

Eguchi Te-No-Hira Ryoji	Technique developed by Toshihiro Eguchi that incorporates palm/hand healing and elements of *Usui-do*.
Eguchi, Toshihiro	Student, friend of Usui-Sensei. Published *Te-no-hira Ryoji Nyumon* (An Introduction to Healing with the Palms) in 1930 and *Te-no-hira Ryoji Wo Kataru* (A Tale of Healing with the Palms of the Hands) in 1954.
Empowerment	Cross-reference: Attunement.
Enkaku Chiryo-Ho	In English: Distant (remote) healing method.

F

Finishing Stroke (also: Nerve Stroke)	Technique from *Usui Shiki Ryoho* Level 2, which is very similar to *Ketsueki Kokan-ho*.
Fire Serpent	Symbol employed within *Raku Kei* Reiki and other modern Reiki traditions. Believed to represent *kundalini* energy that resides within the spine. (Alternately: *Nin Giz Zida*)
Fukuju (Fuku Ju)	Phrase often used as a mantra (or *jumon*) with the mental/emotional symbol. *Fukuju* has been translated to mean: "long and happy life." Or, when used as a toast, it carries an implied meaning of "Cheers!"
Furumoto, Alice Takata	Alice, Takata-Sensei's daughter and Phyllis Lei Furumoto's mother, compiled the 'Gray Book' after Takata's death.
Furumoto, Phyllis Lei	Co-holder of the Office of Grand Master of the Reiki Alliance and Takata-Sensei's granddaughter.

G

Gainen	Term from *Usui-do* that refers to Reiki principles and percepts. *Gainen* = concepts
Gakkai	(In English: Learning society) For example, *Usui Reiki Ryoho Gakkai*.
Gassho	Ritual gesture – place hands together, in front of the mouth, in a prayer-like position. The fingertips rest below the nose. This gesture shows reverence to Bodhisattvas, Buddhas, Teachers, and Patriarchs, and suggests recognition of all beings' oneness.
Gassho Kokyu-Ho	(In English: Gassho breathing method) Breathing through hands as they take the *Gassho* position.
Gassho Meiso	In English: *Gassho* meditation.
Ge Tanden	Energy center located deep inside hara. (Cross-reference: *Seika Tanden*)
Gedoku-Ho	Technique for detoxification, where one hand gets placed at *Seika Tanden*, while the other is placed on lower back at almost the same height.

Gendai Reiki-Ho	(In English: Modern Reiki method) Hiroshi Doi created this modern style of Japanese Reiki that combines elements of traditional Usui technique and teaching with the technique and teaching of complementary energy-healing traditions.
Genetsu-Ho	Technique to bring down high temperature or fever.
Gokai	Five Reiki principles.
Gokai Sansho	Act of reciting the five Reiki principles. *Sansho* = Three times
Gokui Kaiden	*Gendai Reiki-ho* Teacher level.
'Gray Book' ('Grey' Book)	In 1982, Alice Takata Furumoto compiled the 'Gray Book' (Grey Book), which is also known as *Leiki: A Memorial to Takata-Sensei*. This book, featuring excerpts of his writing and Alice's Reiki certificate, was given to Takata's Master Level students.
Grand Master (also: Dai Shihan)	The Reiki Alliance established this title to designate the head of an organization. Also, a loose translation of the term to designate one with the authority to practice Reiki Healing, which is used in certain Japanese Reiki traditions.
Group Reiki	Cross-reference: *Shu Chu Reiki*.
Gumonji-Ho	Also known as Morning Star meditation, which was made popular by the controversial claim that Usui-Sensei was performing this meditation on Kuramayama as he received 'Reiki experience.'
Gyosei (also: Meiji Tenno Gyosei)	Poetry, in a style called *waka*, which was penned by Emperor Meiji. Almost 125 are sung or recited at *Usui Reiki Ryoho Gakkai* meetings.
Gyoshi-Ho	(In English: Gazing method) Healing technique using the eyes.

H

Hado Kokyu-Ho	Technique that involves vocalizing a 'haa' sound as one exhales. Typically used to enhance relaxation. It has been said this vocalization can boost how the immune system functions and elevate vibrational levels.
Hado Meiso-Ho	A *Gendai Reiki-ho* technique of the *hado* breath meditation.

Hamamoto, Kenji	Kenji Hamamoto currently teaches *Hekikuu* Reiki in South Korea, after being based in Sapporo, Japan; this is Hamamoto-san's personal expression and understanding of the healing art, which is based on nearly two decades of practice. His initial Reiki training came from Mieko Mitsui (who also taught Toshitaka Mochizuki and Hiroshi Doi). Then he apprenticed with the Reiki Alliance to study *Usui Shiki Ryoho*. He has also studied with several other Japanese teachers over the years and trained in *Reido* Reiki.
Hand Positions	Positions and placements of hands are important in Reiki healing. Different Reiki traditions employ any of a variety of hand placements or positions for Reiki treatment. Some placement sets include just five positions, while others offer up to twenty.
Hanshin Chiryo-Ho	In English: Half-body treatment method.
Hanshin Koketsu-Ho	(In English: Half-body blood-purifying method) This is a version of the *Ketsueki Kokan-ho* Reiki treatment.
Hara	Term describing the region of the body from the base of the sternum to the top of the pubic bone. The Japanese use this term to describe the seat of an individual's vital power, their *Ki*.
Hara Chiryo-Ho	Cross-reference: *Tanden Chiryo-Ho*.
Hatsurei-Ho	Usui-Sensei is said to have taught this set of, primarily, *Ki-jutsu*-based techniques to enhance self-development. It is more likely that *Hatsurei-Ho* was intended as a ritual where a student receives *reiju*. *Hatsu* = Invoke or generate; *Rei* = Spirit; *Ho* = Method
Hayashi, Chie	Chie received Reiki lessons from her husband Chujiro Hayashi, achieving the Master Level attunement sometime between 1936-37. Born in 1887.
Hayashi, Chujiro	Established the *Hayashi Reiki Ryoho Kenkyukai* after modifying his approach to Reiki with his own understanding of the practice and clinical methodology, around 1930. Hayashi was a student of Usui-Sensei, a retired commander of the Japanese Naval Reserve, and a medical doctor. (1880-1940)

Hayashi Reiki (Ryoho) Kenkyukai	(In English: Hayashi Reiki Treatment Research Association) Founded by Chujiro Hayashi in 1931. After Hayashi's death, Chie, his wife, took over the clinic.
Healing Attunements	Attunement process said to enhance healing process rather than awaken a permanent Reiki ability in the receiver. This is atypical in terms of "normal" Reiki initiation/attunement processes.
Healing Crisis (also: Koten Hanno)	The temporary, cathartic response, or abreaction, some individuals experience during the healing process.
'Healing Space,' The	Cross-reference: Holding the Healing Space.
Hekikuu Reiki	*Hekikuu* ('Azure Sky') Reiki is the tradition established by Kenji Hamamoto based on a personal 'understanding and expression' of Reiki teachings he received over nearly two decades of practice. *Hekikuu* is guided by elements from Japanese 'folk spirituality.'
Heso Chiryo-Ho	Technique that balances energy and benefits the kidneys by applying acupressure from the middle finger directly to the navel.
Hibiki	(In English: Reverberation) A sensation experienced in the hands, which can determine the presence or status of a dis-ease.
Hikari No Kokyu-Ho	(In English: 'Breath of Light' method) A version of *Joshin Kokyu-ho*.
Hikkei	(In English: Companion) In this context, a manual or handbook.
Ho	In English: Technique or method.
Ho	Term from *Gendai* Reiki that refers to Reiki symbols.
'Holding the Healing Space'	Term for process of facilitating a client's 'opportunity for healing.' Meaning, maintaining or creating (i.e., 'holding') a suitable environment – not necessarily physical as much as an emotional or energetic 'environment.' This needs to be a relaxing, safe 'inner space' where an individual could heal themselves from Reiki's energy.

Hon Sha Ze Sho Nen (alternatively: Hon Ja Ze Sho Nen)	Name given to the third Usui Reiki symbol. Considered the 'distant' symbol within Reiki from the Takata lineage (*Usui Shiki Ryoho*). There are some Japanese Reiki traditions, for example, *Hekikuu* Reiki, – where *Hon Sha Ze Sho Nen* is taught as a symbol representing one's mental faculties. This 'symbol' consists of each word: *Hon, Sha, Ze, Sho,* and *Nen*, written in a stylized form of *kanji*. This mantra-type phrase has been translated as: 'Correct Thought (or, mindfulness) is the essence of Being.'

I

Ibuki-Ho	Technique for breathing.
Inamoto, Hyakuten	Received *Jikiden* Reiki teaching from Chiyoko Yamaguchi, teaches a tradition that he has named *Komyo* Reiki, and is an independent Buddhist priest.
Independent Reiki Masters	Term coined in reference to Masters who wanted to pursue Reiki in their own way and do not belong to either the American Reiki Association, Inc. or the Reiki Alliance.
In-Yo	Japanese equivalent to Chinese Yin-Yang.

J

Jaki Kiri Joka Ho	Technique derived from a complex practice named *Ki Barai* and is used for cleansing the energy of *inanimate objects only*.
Japanese Reiki (see also: Western Reiki)	Traditions and styles of Reiki that were established in Japan. These are inherently distinct from the teachings from Takata-Sensei, which are based on *Usui Shiki Ryoho*. Be aware that several Reiki styles classified as Japanese blend both Western and Japanese practice and teachings (for example, *Shinden, Gendai, Reido, Komyo,* and *Vortex*).
Jikiden Reiki	(In English: 'Directly taught' or 'original teaching') Japanese style of Reiki taught by Tadao Yamaguchi. His mother, Chiyoko Yamaguchi, received Reiki instruction from Chujiro Hayashi.
Jiko Joka Ho	A *Gendai Reiki-ho* self-purification practice.
Jisshu Kai	Training/practice meetings.

Jo Tanden (see: Tanden)	Energy center situated between the eyebrows, in the center of the head.
Joshin Kokyu-Ho	Technique focusing on cleansing breath, a *Hatsurei-ho* component, that is employed to purify, stimulate, and strengthen the Reiki flow. This is considered a *Hikari No Kokyu-ho* variant.
Jumon	(In English: A spell, mantra, sacred invocation) Common term for referring to the name of a Reiki symbol (for instance, *Choku Rei* or *Hon Sha Ze Sho Nen*). This indicates the name doubles as a symbol's mantra. Some Reiki traditions have given symbols alternative names, plus a separate mantra that is spoken instead of the symbol's name.

K

Kaicho	(In English: A president or chairman) Title given to the leader of the *Usui Reiki Ryoho Gakkai*.
Kami Tanden (see: Tanden)	Cross-reference: *Jo Tanden*.
Kanji	Chinese characters that are used to write Japanese.
Kanboku	Term used by Yuji Onuki, instructed by Toshihiro Eguchi, to denote Reiki symbols. (Cross-reference: *Shirushi*)
Kantoku	Illuminating visionary state invoked by practicing strict ascetic mystical disciplines that include incantation and mudra-like techniques, meditation, isolation, and fasting.
Karuna Ki	(In English: Compassionate heart energy) Reiki style based on *Tera Mai* and *Karuna* Reiki that was developed by Vincent (Vinny) Amador. Additional elements to *Karuna Ki* have been based on *Raku Kei* Reiki.
Karuna Reiki	Reiki style based on *Sai Baba* Reiki, which was established by William Lee Rand and the International Center for Reiki Training.
Kawamuru, Hawayo	Cross-reference: Takata, Hawayo.
Kenyoku-Ho	(In English: Dry brushing method) Technique for cleansing auras, which is a component of *Hatsurei-ho*.
Kenkyukai	Meetings held by *Usui Reiki Ryoho Gakkai*.

Kenzen No Genri	(In English: Health principles) Book written by Dr. Bizan Suzuki in 1914. It includes a popular admonition: "Today only do not be angry / Do not be afraid / With integrity / Be diligent in your professional duties / Be kind to people." Usui-Sensei might have used this as the direct source for the Reiki *Gokai*, or principles.
Ketsueki Kokan-Ho	(In English: Blood exchange technique) Technique for cleansing blood. Western Reiki uses a version called 'Nerve Stroke' or the 'Finishing' or 'Smoothing' technique.
Kihon Shisei	(In English: Foundation or standard posture) Starting position for *Hatsurei-ho*. Sit in the traditional Japanese *seiza* posture with your eyes closed and your attention focused on *Seika Tanden*.
Ki-Jutsu	(In English: Energetic arts) Term referring to Japanese disciplines that are concerned with developing, strengthening, and refining *Ki*.
Kikai Tanden	Cross-reference: *Seika Tanden*.
Ki Ko	Modern Japanese label for Chinese art of *Chi Gung* (or, *Qi Gong*).
Kiriku	Possible origin of *Sei Heiki*, the second Usui Reiki symbol and 'spiritual emblem' for Amida Butsu.
Koketsu-Ho	In English: Blood-purifying method.
Koki-Ho	(In English: Exhalation method) Healing technique focused on the breath. This is not the same "koki" used in the phrase *Okuden-koki*.
Kokiyu-Ho	(In English: Breath-empowerment method) *Usui Shiki Ryoho* technique used while providing attunement to empower the breath. (Alternately: Sweetening the breath)
Kokoro	Term to refer to the Mind, Will, Heart, and Spirit.
Kokyu-Ho	Technique focusing on breath for developing, strengthening, and purifying *Ki*.

Komyo Reiki	Reiki style that is based on *Jikiden* Reiki, which was developed by Hyakuten Inamoto. Inamoto received Reiki instruction from Chiyoko Yamaguchi. This Reiki style emphasizes *Satori*, or personal spiritual transformation, and pursuing that through Reiki practice. *Komyo* stands on the concept that Usui-Sensei's teachings focused on spiritual development, where any healing was a side effect to spiritual growth.
Koriki	Non-traditional mantra and symbol, called the 'force of happiness' or 'power of happiness,' taught in Level 1 of *Reido* Reiki, is believed to grant serenity and peace.
Koriki	Term that refers to meritous power or spiritual power that is accrued from the practice of numerous venerative, ritual, or meditative disciplines. This term is written with a different *kanji* than the previous entry.
Koshin-Do Mawashi	Term for the Reiki circle method. (Alternatively: Reiki *Mawashi*)
Koten Hanno	Cross-reference: Healing Crisis.
Kotodama	(In English: Word spirit) Multi-faceted discipline based on *Shinto*, of which a primary element involves intoning sacred sounds. This can be both individual vowel sounds and whole syllables.
Kumo	(In English: Cloud) Term employed by some to designate the power symbol. (Cross-reference: *Un* and *Zui-Un*)
Kurama-Yama	Sacred mountain where it is believed that Usui-Sensei first experienced Reiki. *Kurama* = Horse saddle; *Yama* = Mountain

L

Leiki	The spelling of the term Reiki provided in Takata-Sensei's diaries due to there being no true R sound in Japanese.
Leiki: A Memorial to Takata-Sensei	Cross-reference: 'Gray Book.'
Lineage (see also: Reiki Lineage)	Chain of Reiki antecedents going back to Usui-Sensei – your Reiki Teacher, your teacher's Teacher, etc.

| Lotus Repentance Ritual | There is a controversial (due its having no support) claim that Usui-Sensei performed this Buddhist ritual on Kurama-yama as he received the message of the Reiki experience. |

M

Makoto No Kokyu-Ho	(In English: 'Breath of sincerity' or 'breath of truth') Self-development exercise, found in some Reiki styles, taught to enhance awareness of the *Seika Tanden*. Though the claim is that this practice comes from Usui-Sensei's teachings, most likely is that it has been recently borrowed from Aikido.
Master Symbol	Cross-reference: *Dai Ko Myo*.
Matsui, Shou	Wrote what is believed to be the earliest surviving Reiki article in *Nichiyoubi Mainichi* Magazine, from March 4, 1928. Matsui was a student of Chujiro Hayashi, drama teacher, popular playwright, journalist, and advocate for traditional Japanese *Kabuki* Theatre. (1870-1933)
Meiji Tenno Gyo-sei	Cross-reference: *Gyosei*.
Mental/Emotional Symbol	Cross-reference: *Sei Heiki*.
Menkyo Kaiden	(In English: Teacher's license) Certification confirming achievement at the highest levels of proficiency for a specific art. It is said Usui-Sensei gained *menkyo kaiden* at the martial arts school Yagyu Ryu.
Mitsui, Mieko	Mitsui, a Reiki Practitioner and journalist, was the first Practitioner to teach the Western Reiki style in Japan. It has been said he's responsible for sparking the Japanese Reiki revival.
Mochizuki, Toshitaka	Published what is considered to be the earliest modern-day book written by a Japanese Reiki Master in 1995, *Iyashi No Te*. He said some of the historical information came from an obscure Japanese text written by Takichi Tsukida, *The Secret of How to Take Care of Your Family Members*.
Mokunen	(In English: Focus) This is an element of the *Hatsurei-ho* style.
Morning Star Meditation	Cross-reference: *Gumonji-Ho*.

Mugen Muryouju (or: Mugen Muryo Ju)	In an attempt to re-introduce Buddha to Reiki, some Japanese Reiki styles have renamed the SHK symbol to *Mugen Muryouju* or *Muryouju*.
	Muryouju = Japanese name used for Amida Butsu when manifested as the Buddha of Infinite Life; *Mugen* = Infinite wisdom or infinite compassion
Muryouju (Muryo Ju)	Cross-reference: *Mugen Muryouju*.

N

Nade-Te Chiryo-Ho	Using strokes of the hand to stimulate the body's flow of *Ki*.
Nagao, Tatseyi	One of Takata-Sensei's Level 2 students, as reported by Yoshi Kimura, his daughter. It has also been claimed that around 1950 he visited Japan to take Level 3 instruction with Chie Hayashi (Cross-reference: Chujiro Hayashi). Allegedly, he began teaching Reiki when he returned to Hawaii, but none of his students have confirmed this. It is reported that Nagao died in 1980.
Naka Tanden (see: Tanden)	Energy center situated deep within one's chest.
Nao Hi	Cross-reference: *Choku Rei*.
Nentatsu-Ho	Technique taught at Level 1, which is applied to 'realign' habits. Basically, this technique is a type of thought transmission performed with one's hands.
Nerve Stroke (also: Finishing Stroke)	Cross-reference: *Ketsueki Kokan-Ho*.
Nin Giz Zida	Alternate name for 'Fire Serpent' symbol from *Raku Kei* Reiki.

O

Okuden	(In English: Inner teachings) In some Reiki grading systems, this is Level 2. *Oku* = inner; the heart of or depths of a concept; secret or esoteric aspect of a concept.
Okuden Zenki	The first part of the *Okuden* Level within Reiki systems where it is split in two. *-zenki* = First term

Okuden Koki (Okuden Kouki)	The second part of the *Okuden* Level within Reiki systems where it is split in two. -*koki* = Second term
Oshite Chiryo-Ho	(In English: Pressing hand) Technique similar to acupressure, which is applied with pressure from the fingertips.

P

Percepts	Cross-reference: *Gokai.*
Principles	Cross-reference: *Gokai.*
Power Symbol	Cross-reference: *Choku Rei.*

R

Radiance Technique, The	Reiki style Barbara Ray claims was taught to her by Takata-Sensei between 1978-80. This technique incorporates seven Levels or Degrees.
Radiance Technique International Association, Inc., The (RITA)	Founded by Takata-Sensei and Barbara Ray as the American Reiki Association, Inc. in 1980. The RTIA holds Barbara Ray as the legitimate successor to Takata-Sensei's legacy.
Raku	Symbol used in *Raku Kei* Reiki, and Usui/Tibetan Reiki, that resembles an extended lightning bolt. Employed when the attunement process concludes in order to separate the energies and auras of the Teacher from those of the student.
Raku Kei Reiki	Reiki style created by Master Arthur Robertson, which incorporates extra symbols and makes the claim that Reiki has a Tibetan origin. (Alternately: the Way of the Fire Dragon)
Re-attunement	Cross-reference: Repeat Attunement.
Rei	Term meaning to bow. When you bow, you express gratitude, respect, and courtesy for any spiritual being, person, or concept you bow before, and therefore, for yourself as well. This *Rei* is written with a different *kanji* than the word Reiki. *Sensei ni Rei* = Bow to one's Teacher(s) *Shinzen ni Rei* = Bow to a shrine

Reido	(In English: Spirit movement) Involuntary body movements, such as swaying or rocking, which are a type of cathartic response. The application of Reiki or other energy-based therapies may trigger or evoke these types of responses.
Reido Reiki	Japanese Reiki style that tries to combine Japanese traditions with Western Reiki traditions. This system was developed by Huminori Aoki, who is chairman of the Nagoya Reiki Lab.
Reiho (also: Reishiki)	Bowing method, or etiquette.
Reiho	(In English: Spiritual method) For example, *Usui Reiho* = Usui spiritual method. This term is not written with the same *kanji* as the previous entry. For this term, some claim it is a contraction of the phrase Reiki *Ryoho*.
Reiji	(In English: Indication of the Spirit) Spiritual guidance, directed by the knowledgeable placements of one's hands, to provide treatment.
Reiju	Term for original form of Reiki attunement/empowerment. *Rei* = Spiritual; *Ju* = Gift
Reiki	Popular term used to designate the system of healing self-development established by Mikao Usui. Specifically, the term has been applied to denote the therapeutic 'phenomenon' that drives this natural healing process. Recently, this term has achieved a kind of generic status, where it is often being used in reference to any one of the numerous hands-on healing practices, which are typically unrelated to Reiki specifically. Reiki = Spiritual energy, Spiritual feeling, and more accurately, Spirit, Ancestral spirit, Spirit force, Spiritual influence, or Effects of the Spirit in action. (Cross-reference: 'Reiki Consciousness')
Reiki Alliance	Organization formed by several Reiki Masters taught by Takata-Sensei; its purpose was to preserve the integrity of Takata-Sensei's teachings of the *Usui Shiki Ryoho*.
Reiki Circle (also: Reiki Current)	Cross-reference: Reiki *Mawashi*.

'Reiki Conscious-ness'	Term used to denote the perspective that Reiki can be experienced on a deeper level than 'therapeutic energy,' but more on the level of a direct manifestation of a spiritual presence. Either a manifestation of our own spirit or the 'universal' spirit.
Reiki Ethics	Guideline provided to Reiki Practitioners and Teachers outlining ethical and professional conduct.
Reiki (Crystal) Grid	Cross-reference: Crystal Grid.
Reiki Guides	It is believed that they attend to and provide assistance for Reiki Practitioners while they provide treatment. (Alternately: Spirit Beings)
Reiki-Ho	(In English: Reiki method [of healing]) Term used generally as a reference to the Reiki style of healing, and it is used more specifically in reference to *Gendai Reiki-ho*.
Reiki Jutsu	(In English: Art of Reiki) Technically, this term is the name of a martial art that combines elements of *Shotokan* karate with Reiki; it was developed by Andy Wright.
Reiki Lineage	Term to designate the series of Reiki Teachers that exists between a practitioner and Usui-Sensei.
Reikika	Term used for a Reiki Practitioner.
Reiki Marathon	Cross-reference: *Renzoku*.
Reiki Master	A person who has received Master Level attunement, learned how to perform the attunement process at all three levels, held at least one class, and attuned at least one student. (Alternatively: Reiki Teacher)
Reiki Master Practitioner	Term employed within Usui/Tibetan Reiki styles to designate the person who achieved Level 3a. (Cross-reference: Advanced Reiki Training)
Reiki Master Teacher	Term employed within Usui/Tibetan Reiki styles to designate the person who achieved Level 3b. This means a person has been shown the methods for passing Initiation/Attunement and the master symbol. (Cross-reference: Advanced Reiki Training)
Reiki Mawashi	(In English: Reiki Circle; Alternatively: Reiki Current) An energy-cycling meditation performed by a group.

Reiki Ryoho Hik-kei	(In English: Reiki treatment companion) This 68-page, Level 1 manual was compiled by Kimiko Koyama, the *Gakkai*'s sixth *kaicho* and provided to the students of *Usui Reiki Ryoho Gakkai*. Includes: Q&A section, a healing guide, *waka* poetry written by Emperor Meiji, and a Reiki explanation that is believed to be penned by Usui-Sensei personally.
Reiki Ryoho No Shiori	(In English: Guide to Reiki *Ryoho*) Two *Gakkai* presidents, Wanami and Koyama, compiled this document in order to give it to *Usui Reiki Ryoho Gakkai*. *Shiori* encompasses the characteristics of Reiki *Ryoho*, goals for strengthening Reiki, establishing the *Gakkai* administrative system, and the history and purpose of the *Gakkai*. Alongside that, *Shiori* also contains comments from mainstream medical personnel, names for 11 *shinpiden* students of Usui-Sensei, instructions from Usui-Sensei, and various techniques (for instance, *Nentatsuho*, *Byosen*, and *Koketsu-ho*).
Reiki Ryoho To Sono Koka	(In English: *Reiki Ryoho and Its Effects*) Book written in 1919 by Mataji Kawakami. The term Reiki *Ryoho* (In English: Spiritual healing) appears to have been used before Usui-Sensei's time by many therapists who were trying to describe their practice. Note: this book does not explore/explain *Usui Reiki Ryoho*.
Reiki Shower	Technique employed in some Western Reiki styles to cleanse or replenish auras.
Reiki Symbols (see also: Shirushi & Kanboku)	Four tools employed for Reiki Healing. Takata-Sensei teaches that only three should be used by Practitioners during treatments. The fourth symbol is intended to be used for passing attunements to those who want to be Masters.
Reiki Un-Do	Technique where Reiki treatment is received through intentionally initiated spontaneous movement. The *Usui Reiki Ryoho Gakkai*'s sixth *kaicho*, Kimiko Koyama, introduced this method to the society.
Reiki Wa Darenimo Deru	(In English: *Everyone Can Radiate/Emanate Reiki*) A book published privately by Japanese Reiki Master Fumio Ogawa in 1986.

Renzoku | A practice, thought of as a 'Reiki marathon' or 'relay treatment,' where several Practitioners provide Reiki during a single treatment session for a single client. This could last many hours, or even days.

Repeat Attunement (also: Re-attunement) | Western Reiki theory, opposing what Takata-Sensei taught, where repeating attunement could result in a student achieving a deeper connection to Reiki. However, Takata-Sensei believed once a student achieved attunement that it was permanent. Attunement didn't expire, fade, or need a 'topping up.'

Ryoho | (In English: Healing method or medical treatment) For example: *Usui Reiki Ryoho* = Usui Reiki *Treatment*.

Ryoho Shishin | Treatment guide created by Chujiro Hayashi included in Alice Takata Furumoto's 'Gray Book' because Takata-Sensei owned this guide and offered it to some of her students. This guide has similar content to the *Reiki Ryoho Hikkei* healing guide.

S

Sai Baba Reiki | Early version of *Tera Mai* system. (Cross-reference: Kathleen Milner)

Saibo Kassei-Ka | Technique for vitalizing/activating cells based on *Gendai Reiki-ho*.

Saihoji Temple | *Jodo* (meaning, pure land) Buddhist temple in Tokyo where Usui-Sensei's remains are interred, which features a memorial stone installed by members of *Usui Reiki Ryoho Gakkai*.

Scanning | Cross-reference: *Byosen Reikan-Ho*.

Seichim Reiki | Reiki Master Patrick Zeigler established this style, claiming to have spiritual initiation from an Egyptian Sufi order and to have experienced something mystical at the Great Pyramid at Giza.

Seiheki Chiryo-Ho | Technique taught at Level 2, which is a variant of *Nentatsu-ho* that uses Reiki symbols.

Sei Heki (also: Sei Heiki) | (In English: 'Emotional calmness' or 'spiritual composure,' based on *kanji* employed) Name for second Usui Reiki symbol. Referred to as the mental/emotional symbol in Reiki of the Takata lineage (*Usui Shiki Ryoho*). Among Japanese lineages, this symbol is generally known as the 'harmony' symbol.

Seika No Itten	In English: The one point below the navel; Cross-reference: *Seika Tanden*.
Seika Tanden (see: Tanden)	Concept used within traditional Japanese disciplines (artistic, spiritual, or martial), which is generally referred to as *tanden*. This energy center is believed to be almost the same size as a grapefruit and located within the ha-ra. *Seika* = below the navel
Seikaku Kaizen-Ho	(In English: Character improvement method) Another version of, or term for, *Nentatsu-ho*.
Seishin Toitsu	(In English: Unification of mind and spirit) Used as 'Contemplation,' which is an element of *Hatsurei-ho*.
Seiza	A kneeling posture that is traditional to Japan, where a person sits back on or between their heels.
Sekizui Joka Ibuki-Ho	Technique for releasing negativity using *insufflation*, which is described as exhaling energy-breath to release that negativity from the spine. *Sekizui* = Spinal cord; *Joka* = Purification; *Ibuki* = Breath; *Ho* = Method
Sensei	Honorific address that is attached to one's surname by another person (for example, Usui-Sensei). (In English: master, doctor, and more accurately as teacher)
Shashin Chiryo-Ho	Technique for distance healing that employs a picture.
Shihan (also: Shihan Sensei, Dai Shihan)	Term employed in *Jikiden* Reiki for an instructor or Teacher, at the level above *Shihan Kaku*. (In English: An expert who teaches by example)
Shihan Kaku	Term employed in *Jikiden* Reiki for an assistant instructor or Teacher, at the level above *Okuden*.
Shihan Sensei	Cross-reference: *Shihan*.
Shiki	(In English: Style) Used to describe a specific form, version of Reiki, such as *Usui Shiki Ryoho* = Usui *Style* Healing Method.
Shimo Tanden	Cross-reference: *Seika Tanden*.
Shinpiden	(In English: Mystery teachings) In some Reiki grading systems, this is Level 3 (or, Master Level).
Shirushi	(In English: Symbol; Cross-reference: *Kanboku* and Reiki Symbols)
Shoden	(In English: Elementary teachings) In some Reiki grading systems, this is Level 1.
Shu Chu Reiki	Cross-reference: *Shudan* Reiki.

Shudan Reiki	Reiki treatment administered by a group for an individual.
Shuyo-Ho	Version of *Hatsurei-ho* practice that consists of a group.
Sugano, Wasaburo	Chiyoko Yamaguchi's uncle (Cross-reference: *Jikiden* Reiki). In 1928, Sugano received Reiki instruction from Chujiro Hayashi.
Suzuki, Bizan PhD	Cross-reference: *Kenzen No Genri*.

T

Takata, Alice	Cross-reference: Furumoto, Alice Takata.
Takata, Hawayo Hiromi	Reiki Master responsible for bringing the healing practice to the West, born in Hanamaulu, Kauai, Hawaii. Learned Reiki between 1935-38 under Chujiro Hayashi's teachings.
Takata, Saichi	Hawayo Takata's husband, who died in 1930.
Takata-Sensei	(In English: Teacher Takata) This is a respectful title for Hawayo Takata.
Tanden	Energy center, that may be about as big as a grapefruit, which is believed – among Chinese and Japanese philosophies – to exist in 1-3 locations within the body: the abdomen, heart, and/or between the eyebrows. In Japanese, *tanden* is the equivalent of a Chinese term: *tan tien*, which translates to 'field of the elixir.'
Tanden Chiryo-Ho (also: Hara Chiryo-Ho)	Technique to detoxify the body, which is similar to the *Gedoku-ho* technique.
Te-Ate	(In English: Hand treatment) This is a generic term used to designate Japanese healing modalities with hands-on application.
Te No Hira Ryoji Kenkyukai	(In English: Palm Healing Research Society) Toshihiro Eguchi was a student of Usui-Sensei who founded this society.
Tera Mai	Kathleen Milner developed this Reiki system, which was influenced by *Seichim*. Allegedly, Milner received assistance with this process from the Indian spiritual master, Satya Sai Baba.

Therapy	This term has Greek origins in the word *therapeia*, which translates to 'attendance' in terms of providing assistance or help. Generally, Reiki is classified as a therapeutic discipline, even among those who consider it primarily to be a spiritual development system.
Tibetan Master Symbol	Symbol employed in modern styles like *Raku Kei* Reiki. This symbol is considered an equivalent to *Dai Ko Myo*, which is employed within more traditional styles. (Alternatively: *Dumo*)
Tomita, Kaiji	Student of Usui-Sensei who received Reiki instruction around 1925-26. Tomita established the *Tomita Teate Ryohokai* (In English: Tomita Hand-Healing Association) after Usui-Sensei's death, then wrote the book, *Reiki To Jinjutsu – Tomita Ryu Teate Ryoho* (In English: *Reiki and Humanitarian Work – Tomita Ryu Hands Healing*).
Traditional Japanese Reiki (TJR)	Reiki style developed in 1995 by Dave King, which is based on Toshitaka Mochizuki's *Vortex* Reiki. Mochizuki's Reiki style was based on the Radiance Technique.
Traditional Reiki	Term, no longer used, to designate original *Usui Shiki Ryoho* practice that was taught by Takata-Sensei.
Twenty-one-day Cleansing Process	The adjustment period (where the 21 days may correlate with Usui-Sensei's period of austerity from Mount Kurama) some people may experience so the body can absorb the Reiki ability phenomenon. This has been referred to a 'healing crisis' response to receiving attunement and awakening. Though, some people will never experience this 'healing crisis.' Students in the past have been directed to self-treat with Reiki during the adjustment period.

U

Uchite Chiryo-Ho	Palpating or patting technique similar to *Shiatsu*.
Un	(In English: Cloud) Term used as the name for the 'power' symbol. *Kumo* and *Un* are two different ways to pronounce the same *kanji* character. (Cross-reference: *Kumo* and *Zui-Un*)

Un	Term used as the mantra for the 'power' symbol. However, it should not be confused with the previous entry that means 'cloud.' In this case, *Un* is a pronunciation for a Sanskrit 'seed-syllable' mantra that is associated with *Kami Maoson* a deity worshipped by the *Kurama-Kokyo* sect from Mount Kurama.
Usui	(In English: thin) Although it sounds like the surname Usui, this is a term, written in different *kanji*, used by Japanese shamanic practitioners in describing 'power spots.' These are places where the 'veil' is thin between our world and the World of the Spirit.
Usui-Do	(In English: Usui Way) Term referring to Usui-Sensei's original system of spiritual development. Also, a term used by Dave King, and the *Usui-Do Eidan*, to designate a reconstruction of that system.
Usui, Fuji	Usui-Sensei's son (1908-1946).
Usui Kai	(In English: Usui society) Modern term referring to *Usui Reiki Ryoho Gakkai*.
Usui, Kuniji	Usui-Sensei's brother, who worked as a policeman in the area where Usui-Sensei was born – Gifu prefecture.
Usui, Mikao	Creator of the Usui Reiki system of healing and self-development.
Usui Reiki Ryoho (see also: Japanese Reiki)	(In English: Usui Reiki Healing Method) Term that refers to Reiki styles developed in Japan. It is believed this style is most similar to Usui-Sensei's original concept. Utilizes *reiju* versus *denju*, the symbol-centered attunements familiar to Western Reiki. While *Usui Shiki Ryoho* is the more familiar Reiki term, Takata-Sensei also employed the term *Usui Reiki Ryoho*.
Usui Reiki Ryoho Gakkai	(In English: Usui Reiki Healing Method Learning Society) It has been said that Usui-Sensei founded *Usui Reiki Ryoho Gakkai* himself in 1922. However, it is commonly accepted that the society was founded around 1926-27 by Rear Admiral Juusaburo Gyuda (Ushida) and some fellow students.
Usui, Sadako	Usui-Sensei's wife. (Cross-reference: Usui, Mikao)
Usui, Sanai	Usui-Sensei's brother, who was a doctor with a practice in Tokyo or nearby.
Usui-Sensei	(In English: Teacher Usui) The respectful title for Mikao Usui.

Usui Shiki Ryoho (see also: Western Reiki)	(In English: Usui style therapy or Usui style healing method) Western Reiki style taught by Takata-Sensei. This system is divided into three Levels, employing attunements that involve the Reiki symbols.
Usui Teate	(In English: Usui hand treatment) Term used to designate Usui-Sensei's Healing Method.
	However, the term has been selected to designate teachings that are promoted as an expression of Usui-Sensei's spiritual development by Andy Bowling and Chris Marsh. Even more recently, Dave King of *Usui-do* has used this term to designate teachings that are separate even from Bowling's and Marsh's.
Usui/Tibetan Reiki	Reiki style that combines Takata-Sensei's teachings and elements from *Raku Kei* Reiki. It uses a combination of standard Usui Reiki and *Raku Kei* symbols, plus other non-traditional concepts. The third Master Level is typically broken down to 3a and 3b. (Cross-reference: Advanced Reiki Training)
Usui, Toshiko	Usui-Sensei's daughter (1913-1935).
Usui, Tsuru	Older sister of Usui-Sensei.

V

Violet Breath	Technique focused on breath from *Tera Mai* style. (Cross-reference: Breath of the Fire Dragon)
Vortex Reiki	Modern Japanese Reiki style that was developed by Toshitaka Mochizuki. He received instruction from Mieko Mitsui on the Western Reiki style.

W

Waka	(In English: Japanese Song) Short poems that have lines with a fixed number of syllables. The popular Zen haiku is an example of *waka*.
Western Reiki	Term to designate Reiki styles established in the West. For example, *Usui Shiki Ryoho* taught by Takata-Sensei. So, by extension, any Reiki style based on *Usui Shiki Ryoho* would also be considered 'Western.' (Cross-reference: Japanese Reiki)

Y

| Yagyu Ryu | A *Bujutsu* (martial arts) school – founded by Yagyu Muneyoshi Tajima no Kami (1527-1606) – where Usui-Sensei is said to have acquired his *menkyo kaiden* (or, teacher's license), focusing on the arts of *Ju-jutsu* (or, unarmed combat) and *Kenjutsu* (or, swordsmanship). |
| Yamaguchi, Chiyoko | Cross-reference: *Jikiden* Reiki. |

Z

| Zenshin Koketsu-Ho | (In English: Full-body blood-cleansing technique) A version of the *Ketsueki Kokan-ho* technique. |
| Zui-Un | (In English: Auspicious cloud) The phrase translates to 'an omen of good luck.' It had been believed that *Usui Reiki Ryoho Gakkai* did not use names for Reiki symbols. However, it is now believed that they had names all along. |

For instance, they allegedly use this term, *Zui-un*, for the symbol generally called *Choku Rei*. Other Reiki styles have adopted this use of *Zui-un* as well.

(Cross-reference: *Un* and *Kumo*)

FAQS

1. How long does it take to learn Reiki?

The length of time it takes to learn Reiki depends on the Master and the way that they teach the class. It is suggested anywhere between six hours and two days for either Level 1 or the first two levels combined. Enough time to teach and practice giving treatments.

2. Can I learn Reiki myself, or do I need to be initiated?

As stated earlier, while you can teach yourself most of the skills needed for Reiki, you must have an attunement from a Reiki Master to fully embrace the magic and life energy. The flow will not work properly without it. For further reading about the Reiki Attunement ceremony, check out IARP website (at *iarp.org*).

3. How does Reiki positively affect the giver and receiver?

Reiki uplifts and energizes both parties during the process. Even if the receiver is skeptical at first, they will usually leave the session much more balanced, happier, and with a positive sense of well-being. Givers become more aware of their own energetic state and notice an uplift in it once a session is over, which has a roll-over effect.

4. How does Reiki help you become your best self?

The key thing to understand about Reiki or any other energy healing modalities is how energy is related to our overall health. Dis-ease of the body actually stems from the energetic body first then appears in our physical body the last, so if we want to find out the root cause of what's going on with our health, we must look into what our energetic state is like and start taking responsibility of our own thoughts and actions.

What this means is Reiki makes us take notice of our energy flow and what is affected by it. Our physical, emotional, and spiritual state, and by taking onboard the five Reiki principles, we make a positive change to any negativity that we notice within ourselves, becoming the best version of ourselves.

5. How do I protect myself from taking other people's negativity on when performing a Reiki session?

While it is unlikely that you will ever take on anyone else's negativity, while performing Reiki, as it always concentrates more on the positive, you can still protect yourself if you choose by making sure you go in with the right intention. You may think: *"I ask for protection and assistance from my guides, angels, and Spirit as I offer this Reiki session."* You can also visualize blue, gold, and white in your aura, allowing only positive energy to enter.

6. How can I become a strong Reiki healer?

The best way to become a strong Reiki healer is to practice your skills every single day to strengthen your intuition and also to understand the flow a little better. But you can also self-attune to ensure that you are fully in touch with your Reiki and also that it's the strongest it can be.

7. What are the disadvantages of using Reiki?

There aren't many disadvantages to using Reiki, but **here is a list of a few things that you should be aware of before starting** on this journey:

- No formal regulation. While there are organizations that Reiki practitioners can belong to, there isn't a regulatory body.

- Limited science. Right now, there aren't enough scientific studies or funding to 'prove' its effectiveness, which can put some people off.

- Because of the lack of science, not many health insurance companies will fund the treatments. Shop around to ensure this if it's something you need.

- Variation. Everyone reacts differently because everyone has individual things that need treating, so no one can guarantee how you will feel after.

8. What do I do if I feel my Reiki diminishing?

If, over time, you feel your Reiki energy beginning to deplete, there is likely some blockage in your emotional chakras that needs to be cleared. The best way to do this is to be persistent, to keep practicing, and to also ensure that you keep up your mindful meditation until the blockage is cleared.

9. What do I do if I feel weak after a Reiki session?

There is always a chance that you will feel weak after a Reiki session, which can last for moments, hours, or even days. This is known as the 'healing crisis.' You can try to avoid it by drinking at least four 8-ounce glasses of water within the two hours before the session and you can plan to rest afterward, but you may not be able to avoid it.

You need to listen to your body. If you crave something, have it; if you need rest, take it. Reiki is looking after you long after the session has ended, so whatever you feel like you need, you do. Even if you haven't realized it before.

10. How do I help rid others of negativity with Reiki?

Perform your Reiki with the intention of getting rid of negativity and use the Reiki symbols to strengthen your energy flow to make sure you're at the highest energy vibration to assist you with this. For further reading, check out Reiki Web (at *www.reikiwebstore.com*).

11. What is the usual cost of Reiki treatment?

It is suggested that Reiki sessions generally cost around $50 to $75 dollars a session. Students may offer a lower fee as they train, and some Reiki clinics offer community circles for a low fee.

12. How is healing myself different from healing others?

It isn't any different to heal someone else to yourself, aside from the hand positions. Your intention may be different, but the way that your energy flows will be very similar, changing only due to the need for the Reiki.

13. Who can perform a distance healing and how?

As soon as you are Level 2 in your Reiki training, you can begin sending distance Reiki using the *Hon Sha Ze Sho Nen* symbol. Anyone can do this once they have learned how to heal others. You need to channel your energy and send it to the right place with the intention to make this happen. You can **read a full guide for doing this** from Reiki (at *www.reiki.org/reikinews/distanthealing.htm*).

- Picture who you are sending Reiki energy to. Have the clear intention to send Reiki energy at each level of being for around 10-20 minutes.

- Visualize the Reiki energy entering that person's crown chakra to project to the physical level of being. Then, it can enter their body to gently and slowly fill them up. As the Reiki energy fills them up, all their organs and parts will be infused with Reiki. This is when the energy will begin to radiate out. Visualize them glowing from this healing energy. You might see them expanded because their first energy layer has been filled.

- Next, you can project Reiki to the emotional being. Visualize them being filled with contentment, peace, love, joy, and overall well-being.

Now picture that glow from their physical body extending out to expand their emotional level.

- Then, project the Reiki energy to the mental being. Imagine their thoughts being calm and clear. Visualize their brain working so well that thoughts flow easily. Intend that solutions to perplexing problems will be well thought out. Picture worry gently flowing away from their physical being. As these stressful thoughts leave their being, Reiki energy fills them up and expands the mental level.

- Next, you can project Reiki energy to the spiritual being. Visualize Reiki energy filling up and restoring their spirit, essence, and soul. See it like a glowing river of energy with a direct link to higher realms. Picture guidance flowing in, that this person is directly connected to the higher realms or whatever source they rely upon. Direct the Reiki energy so that it relights the flame, so that it reconnects them to the inner divine. Imagine spiritual energy extending out beyond any other level of this being.

- Try simply having an in-depth conversation with this person before you project any Reiki energy. This would allow you to address every level of their being before starting the session. For their physical body, ask if they are feeling any pain or discomfort. For their emotional body, ask if there is something specific triggering a specific emotion. For their mental body, ask if there is something weighing on their mind or if there is a specific worry or doubt. For their spiritual body, ask if they recognize the sacredness within everyday life or if they feel isolated or unprotected within the world.

- Before you begin, ask them to open themselves up to the Reiki energy that can heal all the levels of their being. They need to allow themselves to be open to receive the healing energy.

- Send healing Reiki energy for about 10-20 minutes toward each level of being. Direct the Reiki toward the feelings, thoughts, or issues that were discussed.

- After completing the session, tell them to rest. Picture a power symbol, then seal the session with love and light. Perform *Kenyoku* (dry bathing) to disconnect from their field of energy. Perform Reiki on yourself for a few minutes. Consider calling them afterwards to hear about their experience and share your own.

14. Does Reiki help clean an aura, and what are the best aura-cleansing exercises?

Reiki clears all blockages and negative energies, and that includes your aura. If your Reiki is needed there, then that's where it will work. But if this is a real issue for you and you need more, here are some **aura-cleaning exercises**:

- Take a sea salt bath or use Himalayan salt stones with the intention of cleaning your aura.
- Visualize, using meditation, five to ten minutes a day.
- Use a sage smudge to clear your aura.
- Try a selenite wand to draw out the negative energy blocks.
- Use the wind or sunlight to clear the blockages.
- A chime with a nice resonant ring will help.

15. *How do I find, connect, and awaken Higher and Divine Self with the help of Reiki techniques and meditation?*

Reiki helps you to connect with your Higher and Divine Self by driving you towards the best version of you simply by noticing. The more you practice this new skill, the more you will connect. The same goes for meditation.

16. *Is Reiki effective for animals, children, and the elderly?*

Yes! Reiki can be effective on any living thing. There are no limits to who you can help, and that includes animals, children, and the elderly. This can be done using the hand positions or distance healing; there are no limits.

CONCLUSION

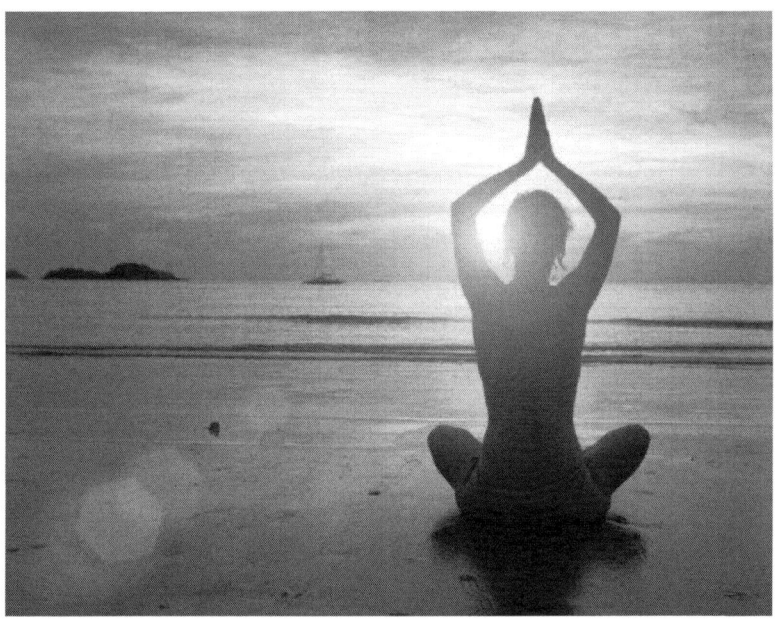

So, now that you have seen how easy it is to learn Reiki and the benefits that you and your loved ones can get from it, why not give it a try? You could start with a session, then go on to have a class and an attunement to get hold of the energy flow yourself.

Then, the possibilities are endless.

Not only will you be given a new skill to help you feel happier and have a fulfilling life, with better balance and a healthier well-being, you can also help others too – maybe even gaining a way to make money.

Just in case you need reminding, here are **ten benefits of Reiki**:

- Relieves stress and tension, relaxing your muscles.

- Reducing pain and soreness.
- Getting rid of negative energy blocks, giving you a clearer mind. Also helping you to love yourself.
- Stop you from immediately jumping to negative reactions.
- Sharpens intellect.
- Mends relationships by rekindling love and applying some empathy.
- Assists success, especially when sent to a moment of importance in the future.
- Sharpens our sixth sense.
- Brings balance to our lives and helps us to overcome past trauma.
- Reestablishes the psychical, emotional, spiritual, mental, and professional to bring everything into alignment.

You have everything that you need to get started with Reiki now, mostly because the majority of it is already inside of you, it's time to get started. There are some additional resources at the end of this book to give you more to work with.

Good luck on your Reiki journey!

USEFUL RESOURCES

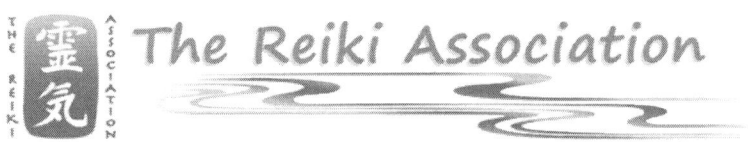

www.reikiassociation.net

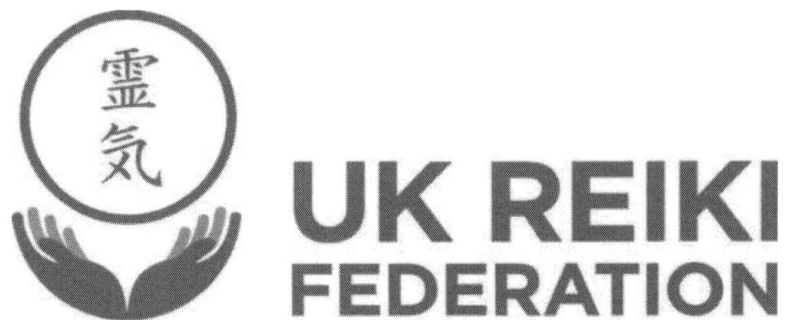

www.reikifed.co.uk

.THE INTERNATIONAL CENTER.

— *for* —

REIKI
TRAINING

www.reiki.org

www.holisticshop.co.uk/dictionary/healing-reiki

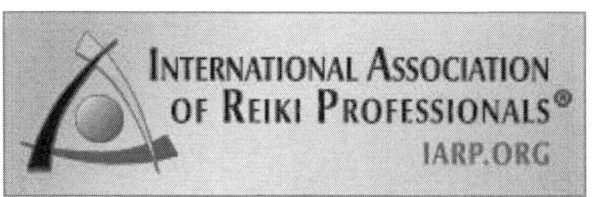

iarp.org

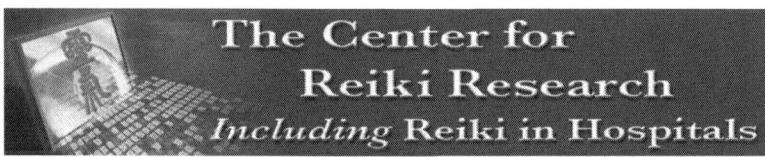

www.centerforreikiresearch.org

ABOUT THE AUTHOR

Karen Gray is a Reiki Master, intuitive energy healer, and mindfulness expert. She has devoted her life to the study of energy and alternative healing techniques, including sound healing, metaphysical healing, Feng Shui, and crystal healing. Gray believes that the key to a healthy body is an attuned mind and soul, and practices meditation and mindfulness herself to maintain spiritual, emotional, and physical health. She teaches classes and runs workshops throughout the United States in all the subjects she studies, and is dedicated to spreading information and awareness about spiritual health to all. These practices have transformed every aspect of Gray's life – and so, it is her life's calling to bring that transformation to others. Her teachings are for anyone who searches to calm their mind, ground themselves in the present, and find joy in the life they are living.

Printed in Great Britain
by Amazon

53393652R10079